THE LYMPHOEDEMA HANDBOOK

Causes, effects & management

Professor Neil B. Piller
&
Maree O'Connor P.T.

HILL OF CONTENT

Disclaimer

This book is not intended to be used as a substitute for professional health care and assistance. While every effort has been made to provide accurate and reliable information, the authors and publisher cannot be held responsible for any consequences of applying the facts and advice presented.

First published in Australia 2002
by Hill of Content Publishing Pty Ltd
86 Bourke Street, Melbourne 3000
Tel: 03 9662 2282
Fax: 03 9662 2527
Email: hocpub@collinsbooks.com.au

Reprinted 2002

Cover design: D Snibson, Modern Art Production Group
Typesetting: Midland Typesetters, Maryborough
Printed in Australia by McPherson's Printing Group

National Library Cataloguing-in-publication data

The lymphoedema handbook: causes, effects & management.

Bibliography.
ISBN 0 85572 327 0

1. Lymphoedema – Popular works. 2. Lymphoedema – Treatment –
Popular works. I. Piller, N.B. (Neil B.), 1951–.
II. O'Connor, Maree, 1967–.

616.42

THE LYMPHOEDEMA HANDBOOK

Causes, effects & management

Contents

Co-authors

Tammy Boatman, occupational therapist
Mercy Lymphoedema Clinic, Austin and Repatriation Medical Centre, Melbourne, Victoria, Australia

Rosalind Deacon, physiotherapist
John Lindell Rehabilitation Unit, Anne Caudle Campus, Bendigo Health Care Group, Bendigo, Victoria, Australia

Eric Haan, Associate Professor and clinical geneticist
South Australian Clinical Genetics Service, Women's and Children's Hospital, North Adelaide, South Australia, Australia

David McCombe, plastic surgeon
St Vincent's Hospital, Bernard O'Brien Institute of Microsurgery, Melbourne, Victoria, Australia

Maree O'Connor, physiotherapist
Victorian Lymphoedema Practice, Melbourne, Victoria, Australia

Wayne A. Morrison, Professor of Surgery and Director
The University of Melbourne, Department of Surgery, St Vincent's Hospital, Bernard O'Brien Institute of Microsurgery, Melbourne, Victoria, Australia

Neil Piller, Professor, team leader and clinical research scientist
Lymphoedema Assessment Clinic, Flinders Surgical Oncology and Department of Public Health, School of Medicine, Flinders University, South Australia, Australia

Hildegard Reul-Hirche, physiotherapist
Royal Brisbane Hospital & Royal Women's Hospital and Health Service Districts, Queensland, Australia

Terence Ryan, Professor of Dermatology
Oxford Centre for Health Care, Research and Development, Oxford Brookes University, Oxford, United Kingdom

Penelope Sanderson, social worker
Mercy Lymphoedema Clinics, Mercy Hospital for Women, Melbourne, Victoria, Australia

Louis Vecchié, dietitian
Mercy Hospital for Women, Melbourne, Victoria, Australia

Christopher Wheeler, podiatrist
Brunswick Foot Clinic, Melbourne Foot Clinic, Melbourne, Victoria, Australia

Acknowledgements

A book like this could not have come together without the expertise, time and energy of a number of people whose contributions were generously given without remuneration. The Lymphoedema Association of Victoria Inc especially wishes to thank the health professionals who contributed to the text: the dedicated principal authors Maree O'Connor and Neil Piller; and specialist contributors Tammy Boatman, Rosalind Deacon, Eric Haan, David McCombe, Wayne Morrison, Hildegard Reul-Hirche, Terence Ryan, Penelope Sanderson, Louis Vecchié and Christopher Wheeler. Sincere thanks are also due to Adrienne Anstee and Liz Dart for their invaluable input: Liz for helping get the project up and running; and Adrienne for so successfully seeing the project through. We also thank Nola and Geoff Brown for sharing so eloquently their personal experience of lymphoedema. Finally, the Lympoedema Association of Victoria Inc gratefully acknowledges the generous financial support of The International Ladies Group Inc.

Foreword

Around 250,000 Australian men and women have or are at risk of contracting lymphoedema, which can develop when the body's lymphatic system fails or is overloaded. While lymphoedema is not life-threatening it can produce unwelcome symptoms, including swelling of the limbs, and have a considerable impact on the patient's quality of life.

The Lymphoedema Association of Victoria Inc (Australia) has for some time felt the need for an inexpensive and user-friendly guide for lymphoedema patients and their families, carers and health professionals. It was generally agreed that people currently working in the field were best placed to provide the necessary information. This book therefore brings together contributions from a number of committed professionals who have a special interest in lymphoedema within their own discipline, chief of whom are the co-authors: physiotherapist Maree O'Connor and clinical research scientist Neil Piller. Liz Dart (former Secretary of the Lymphoedema Association of Victoria) and Adrienne Anstee (Anti-Cancer Council Victoria), also brought their personal experience to bear in developing the framework and author guidelines.

As with many medical conditions, the sooner lymphoedema is diagnosed and treated the better the outcome. This book describes simply but informatively the lymphatic system, the signs and symptoms of lymphoedema, diagnostic techniques, and current forms of management and treatment. And, perhaps just as importantly, it also looks realistically at the psychological and lifestyle challenges which often accompany lymphoedema.

Lymphoedema often affects not only the patients themselves but also their families, friends and even work colleagues. This book is written for the general community and health professionals. It is hoped that it will help everyone involved better understand lymphoedema, its management and treatment.

PART 1

The Lymphatic System

This section explains the lymphatic system. Chapter 1 summarises our still-developing understanding of the structure and function of this vital network. Chapter 2 looks at the condition lymphoedema, which occurs when there is a blockage somewhere in the lymphatic system and is characterised by swelling and other symptoms.

ONE

About the lymphatic system

The lymphatic system – like that other important network with which it is closely linked, the vascular system or bloodstream – transports fluid around the body. Specifically, it collects and carries excess fluid (lymph) and other material from body cells and tissues, filters out larger particles such as bacteria and then delivers the fluid back into the bloodstream. In this way it plays an important part in protecting the body from disease.

How the lymphatic system works

Lymphatic vessels are distributed all over the body, alongside arteries and veins. At certain points they meet a knot of tissue known as a lymph node (or lymph gland), where foreign particles are filtered out and protective antibodies and white blood cells (lymphocytes) are collected. It is estimated that there are between 25 and 60 lymph nodes in the armpit alone, although some of these are very small.

In normal conditions the lymphatic system pumps 2–4 litres of lymph each day, though the flow rate and volume may vary. If lymph nodes are removed, damaged or destroyed (during surgery, for example), lymph drainage is reduced.

Ultimately the lymph vessels join together to form two large ducts, the thoracic duct and the right lymphatic duct, which drain into veins near the heart (Figure 1.1). The tonsils, spleen and thymus are part of the lymphatic system.

The fluid percolating around the spaces between body cells carries nutrients and oxygen, which all cells need to survive. Most of this fluid goes straight back into the blood vessels. Fluid is mainly carried into the lymphatic system by the small vessels

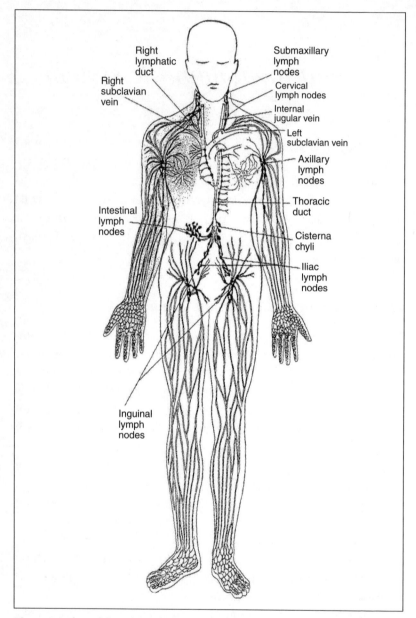

Figure 1.1 If you follow the paths these larger lymphatic vessels take from the extremities, you will see that those from both legs, the left side of the torso, and the head and the left arm drain into the blood system near the left collarbone. The vessels from the right side of the torso and head and the right arm drain into the blood system near the right collarbone.

known as lymphatic capillaries, as the result of variations in pressure that occur as the body moves and muscles contract and relax. The fluid is then pushed onto larger vessels (lymphatics), which pulsate rhythmically – usually at the rate of 6–10 beats per minute – in response to the amount of fluid waiting to be removed (Figure 1.2). They will beat faster if there is more fluid to be carried, and in response to particular actions (such as gentle exercise) and some medications.

Some lymph vessels have small valves which help propel the lymph forwards and ensure that it flows in one direction only. The flow of lymph in the upper part of the limbs may also be affected by respiratory movements: taking deep breaths can help lymph pass into the larger lymph vessels in the chest area and so help drainage into the blood system.

Each lymphatic vessel has enormous reserve capacity. The normal load is usually only about one-tenth of the vessel's transport capacity, which means that most of the time these vessels are just 'idling'. But sometimes the lymph load is greater than the vessel's transport capacity, and this causes swelling (lymphoedema).

Research into the lymphatic system

Compared to blood vessels, lymphatics are thin-walled and very fragile. When touched they constrict into fine thread-like

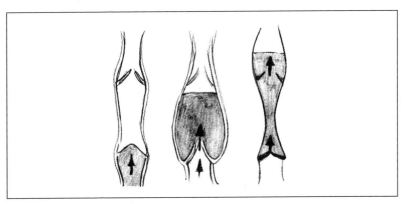

Figure 1.2 The movement of lymph through lymph vessels showing the pumping unit of the lymph system called the lymphangion.

structures, and they are often obscured by fat in the tissues. Lymph itself is a clear, watery fluid which is only visible to the naked eye when it accumulates in a blister. For these reasons the lymphatic system is difficult to see, even for surgeons, and has been difficult to study. Our understanding of it therefore lags far behind what we know about the blood system.

As early as 300 BC, the Greek physicians Erasistratus and Herophilus described the lymphatic vessels which drained the abdominal area after a person had eaten a fatty meal (the lymphatics absorb fat, which turns the normally clear lymph white). Although their description was not entirely accurate (they called the vessels 'arteries' and thought that the fluid in them was white blood), it was a good start. However, it was not until about 1550 AD that Eustaceous identified the thoracic duct and traced its path through the chest.

In the 1620s, the Swede Olaus Rudbeck traced the course of most of the body's lymphatic vessels and showed that this network was really a second circulatory system. Around the same time, Gaspar Aselli in Italy discovered the very fine lymphatic vessels (lymphatic capillaries), which were named by Thomas Bartholin in 1653. Much of their work was preserved and is stored at Siena University in Italy and at the University of Uppsala in Sweden.

There were further developments in the eighteenth century, when William Hunter, William Hewson and William Cruikshank not only clarified the anatomy of the lymphatic system but also described its basic functions in some detail. Since then, people such as Ernest Starling, Cecil Drinker, John Kinmonth, Michael Földi and John Casley-Smith have all added details to our knowledge, but there are now very few researchers undertaking further investigations.

The main drainage pathways

Through the work of Anton Kubic and Michael Földi, we know that the lymphatic system consists of a series of territories separated by boundaries called watersheds. There are four main territories in the torso, four in each leg and six in each arm (three each in the forearm and upper arm (Figures 1.3 and 1.4).

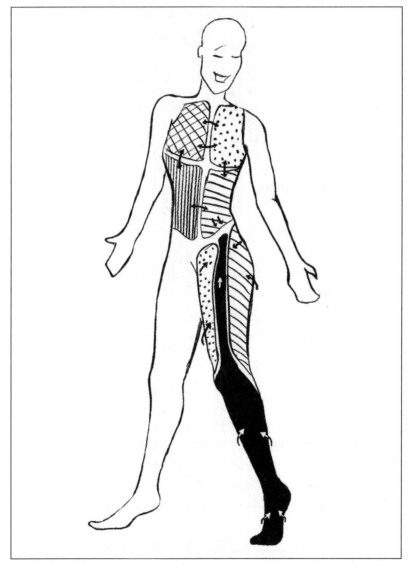

Figure 1.3 There are four major lymph territories of the torso and each leg. Only three major ones of the leg are shown here; the other is behind in the calf area. The arrows show the direction of normal lymph drainage.

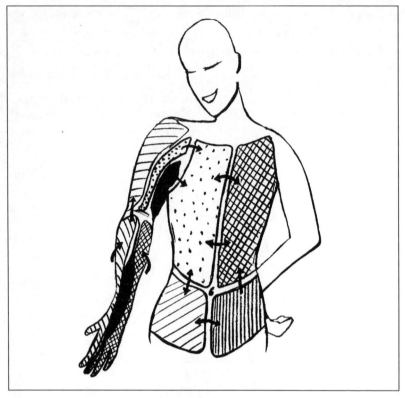

Figure 1.4 There are six major lymph territories for each arm, three for the forearm and three for the upper arm. The arrows show the direction of normal lymph drainage.

As shown in Figure 1.5, the lymphatic system in a limb is basically a two-level network comprising a deep system (the larger vessels) and a superficial system (the smaller vessels).

There are 20–30 larger lymphatic vessels (lymph collectors) in the forearm, combining into about half this number in the upper arm (Figure 1.6). 2–4 of these collectors typically pass to the outer side of the arm and are thus usually spared surgery or radiotherapy damage.

There are 15–25 larger vessels on the upper surface of the foot, which similarly combine into between 5–10 in the lower leg. The upper leg has between 10–20 larger lymphatic vessels. Near the inner part of the knee there is a 'bottleneck' where most of

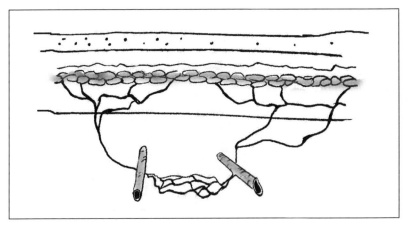

Figure 1.5 The lymphatic system is a two-level network.

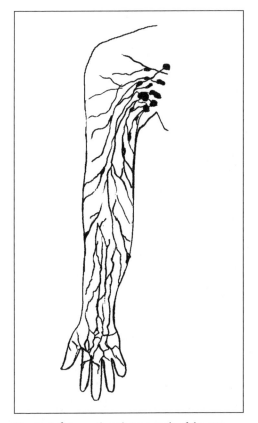

Figure 1.6 Larger lymphatic vessels of the arm.

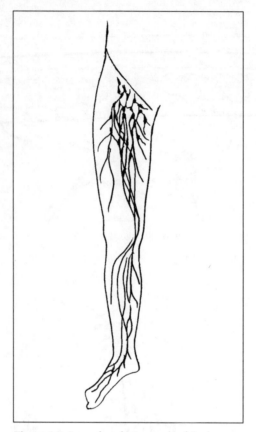

Figure 1.7 Larger lymphatic vessels of the leg.

the lymphatic vessels from the lower limb come close together. Any damage to this area may jeopardise drainage from the whole lower leg (Figure 1.7).

When the lymphatic system fails

If a lymphatic territory becomes blocked because the system has failed to remove the normal load of fluid, the area drained by it will swell. This is the condition known as lymphoedema. If the blockage is near the top of an arm or leg, territories further away may also suffer a build-up of lymph. In this event, some action or treatment is needed to help the system function properly again. A blocked territory can, for example, be helped to drain by opening up pathways across watersheds to other territories (by massage, for example). This is the basis of many of the treatments described in Part 2 of this book.

When there is a build-up of lymph, some cells in the affected tissue may also fail to function properly. This is commonly the case with macrophages, white blood cells which help protect the body from disease and keep body tissue in good condition (for more information, see the section 'Associated Changes and Conditions' on page 19).

TWO

Lymphoedema

As outlined in Chapter 1, lymphoedema is a swelling caused by failure of the lymphatic system to remove a normal load of protein and fluid from body tissues. Swelling can even occur when the lymph system is normal, but is greatly overloaded. Once acquired, lymphoedema is a lifelong condition, but it is not life-threatening and can in most cases be greatly improved by treatment.

Lymphoedema can occur because of some malformation or poor development of the lymphatic system, which may be present at birth (genetically inherited) or arise much later (most typically around puberty or age 30–40). These are referred to as primary lymphoedemas, which according to the most recent research account for 5–10 per cent of all lymphoedemas.

The lymphatic system may also fail as a consequence of surgery or radiotherapy which removes or destroys lymph vessels and nodes, or because tumours or other structures are pressing on the delicate vessels, or owing to inflammation within the vessels themselves (lymphangitis). This is known as secondary lymphoedema. Research indicates that about 30 per cent of women who have treatment for breast cancer which involves removal of lymph glands will develop this swelling, as will about 30 per cent of men and women who have lymph glands removed during treatment for reproductive system or bowel cancers. It is suggested that up to another 30 per cent will have added symptoms such as heaviness, tension, aches and pains in the limb on the side where treatment takes place. Based on estimates from Australia and overseas, around 250,000 Australian men and women have or are at risk of having these problems.

Not all swellings are lymphoedemas

Any accumulation of fluid which results from a change to the vascular system and causes body tissue to swell is called oedema; this is a fairly common condition.

It is important to be aware of other factors which may contribute to lymphoedema or other conditions which may look like it. For example, following a spider or insect bite the surrounding area or perhaps a whole limb may swell for a few days because additional fluids and proteins escape from the bloodstream and enter the spaces between the cells. Once the surplus material is removed by the lymphatic system and macrophages, the swelling goes down.

There are many other circumstances and conditions that may result in oedema. For example, surgery may produce temporary oedema when more than a normal amount of fluid leaks from blood vessels due to the surgical process. Also, high blood pressure can result in excess leakage from blood capillaries as the higher pressure forces more fluids out of the small gaps between the cells. Sometimes the vascular system does not function normally, because blood vessels are abnormally fragile (weak) or abnormally dilated (varicose), are clotted (thrombosis) or inflamed, or because valves are defective. The resulting condition, called phlebo-lymphoedema, hinders the reabsorption of fluids by the blood vessels. It is important to treat any such oedema conditions, because they put an increased load on the lymphatic system.

Other parts of the body may influence what happens in a limb. For instance, an underactive thyroid can also result in a form of oedema called myxoedema. There are other conditions involving more localised fluid accumulations as the result of other endocrine system disorders, but these are rare. The condition called lipoedema, which is almost exclusively restricted to women, is a problem related to increased formation of fatty tissue (hyperplasia), especially in the hips and thighs and often extending to the ankles; it has a genetic basis. In severe cases, the distribution of fat may impair lymphatic drainage, in which case it may be called *lipo-lymphoedema*; sufferers generally (but not always) have skin that is painful to the touch, even with light pressure.

Primary lymphoedema

Primary lymphoedema results from abnormal development of the lymphatic system before birth and occurs most commonly where there is a family history of the condition. It should, however, be stressed that people will not necessarily develop lymphoedema just because their parents or grandparents did.

GENETIC INFLUENCES

Genes provide the chemical blueprint for normal development, growth and everyday functioning of the body. In all individuals, one in each pair of genes is inherited from the mother and the other from the father. Both of the genes in each pair are usually normal, but sometimes there is an error in the genetic code of one or both genes in a pair.

DIFFERENT FORMS OF PRIMARY LYMPHOEDEMA

Lymphoedema is said to be congenital if it is present at birth or develops soon thereafter, juvenile if it begins around puberty (sometimes referred to as *Lymphoedema praecox*), and adult if it begins during adulthood (sometimes referred to as *lymphoedema tarda*). The onset of the juvenile and adult forms is sometimes associated with an infection or injury, but often no triggering factor can be identified.

When primary lymphoedema occurs in association with some other condition, such as hypo-parathyroidism (an underactive parathyroid gland which causes low blood calcium levels), it is said to be syndromic.

Congenital lymphoedema (known as hereditary lymphoedema type 1 or Nonne–Milroy lymphoedema) was first described in 1865. Research suggests that faults in hereditary lymphoedema type 1 is usually caused by faults in the FLT4 gene on chromosome 5, but it is known that at least one other, as yet unknown, gene can cause the disorder. Most commonly inherited, this form of lymphoedema affects males and females equally. It usually occurs in the legs only (typically affecting both limbs with equal severity), but the genitalia and even the face and upper limbs are sometimes involved. Its incidence is estimated to be 1 in 6000 births, which makes it one of the more common genetic disorders of childhood. The basic problem is that the major lymphatic vessels fail to develop and there is also little or no development of alternative pathways.

Juvenile lymphoedema (hereditary lymphoedema type 2, or Meige lymphoedema) was described in 1898. It is also dominantly inherited, but differs from the congenital form in affecting about twice as many girls as boys and commonly involving one leg more than the other or one leg only. It is thought to be more common than congenital lymphoedema, but precise figures are not available. No gene has yet been identified as being responsible for this form of lymphoedema, but, as with type 1 it is likely that at least one gene can cause the problem. Not everyone who inherits a gene for juvenile lymphoedema will go on to develop it: about 80–85 per cent do so, although those who never develop the disorder can still pass it on to their children.

There are several forms of *syndromic lymphoedema*, which is when lymphoedema occurs in connection with some other disorder. Congenital lymphoedema can, for example, occur with hypoparathyroidis, microcephaly (an abnormally small head and brain), intestinal lymphangiectasia (an unco-ordinated overgrowth of lymph vessels) or with mental retardation (Hennekam syndrome). In school-age children, lymphoedema can occur with cholestasis (blocked bile flow, also called Aagenaes syndrome). In teenagers, it can occur with distichiasis (a double row of eyelashes) or with vascular malformations of the brain; in adults, it may accompany yellow nail syndrome (see 'Toenails', page 88). Each of these conditions has a genetic basis and presumably the gene involved contributes in some way to the lymphatic disorder.

Secondary lymphoedema

Anyone who undergoes surgery and/or radiotherapy to the breast, armpit, pelvis or groin, or experiences any other episode that damages or destroys lymphatic vessels or nodes, could develop secondary lymphoedema. But not everyone in these circumstances will do so and the risk generally depends on age, the side on which the surgery took place (related to hand dominance), the number of vessels and/or nodes removed, whether or not the patient undergoes radiotherapy, and body mass. The chance of lymphoedema is lower (about 5 per cent) when a small number of lymph nodes are removed and no radio-therapy treatment is given in that area. The risk increases to about 30 per cent when a large number of lymph nodes are removed and radiotherapy is given to those remaining.

Each person has a slightly different lymphatic system in terms of the number and location of lymph vessels and the pathways they take. This is one reason why it is difficult to make an accurate assessment and to predict whether or not a person will develop lymphoedema after surgery or radio-therapy. In some cases even a large amount of damage to part of the lymphatic system will not result in lymphoedema, whereas in others even a small wound or other problem may precipitate the condition. It is therefore important that a health practitioner has the fullest possible medical, surgical and family details of each patient.

Even when a condition that overloads the lymphatic system is present, fluids will not accumulate unless the system's reserve capacity is exceeded. In someone born with insufficient lymph vessels, the existing vessels will take on the extra load. They may handle this easily, in which case lymphoedema will not develop, whereas if the load is too great lymphoedema may appear temporarily during bouts of strenuous activity or in the presence of an infection. Sometimes the superficial (smaller) lymphatics will take over the work of the larger ones, but they can only handle a correspondingly smaller volume of lymph. If vessels are unable to carry the waiting lymph load, lymphoedema will eventually become chronic.

Once larger lymph vessels are severed, they are unlikely to regenerate. The smaller vessels (lymphatic capillaries) can do so, a fact that can be exploited in treatment strategies such as laser treatment and frictional massage, which help to slightly break up the structure of the tissues. However, no lymphatic vessel can grow through scar tissue – even 0.5 mm of scar tissue will prevent growth – so it is important to minimise the formation of scar tissue and to facilitate the removal of any that does form.

The published statistics on the incidence of arm and leg lymphoedema vary widely. Some patients develop lymphoedema after apparently minor surgery (such as the stripping of varicose veins), possibly because some lymph vessels have inadvertently been removed along with the vein. A recent Australian survey showed that secondary lymphoedema does not always develop immediately after surgery or radiotherapy, but takes an average of 3½ years to become apparent. (This research focused on arms, but the timing is likely to be similar for legs). However, in many cases, lymphoedema can occur earlier or later than that and timely attention to the limb (see Chapter 3) may reduce the risk of lymphoedema developing.

Signs and symptoms of lymphoedema

While it is extremely difficult to predict if and when lymphoedema might occur, there are indicators that a person may be at risk. The symptoms summarised below may occur in all or part of the limb or in the breast (or adjacent chest area) following a mastectomy or lumpectomy and axillary clearance (when lymph nodes are removed from the armpit) with or without radiotherapy. A groin clearance (removal of lymph nodes from the groin) and associated radiotherapy may produce symptoms in the genital or lower abdominal area. The main signs of possible risk include:

- a swelling that comes and goes with exercise or other physical activity
- feelings of heaviness, pain or tension in the limb
- a 'bursting' feeling (tightness and fullness) in the limb
- pins and needles
- numbness
- redness and a sensation of heat

If a limb begins to feel warm and becomes red, this may signal the infection often called cellulitis or erysipelas (see page 20). It is sometimes referred to as lymphangitis, although this is really a bacterial inflammation of lymph vessels. Any symptoms of warmth and redness in a limb should be investigated as soon as possible, as early treatment is essential.

Some of these symptoms might be a natural after-effect of surgery or radiotherapy, and lymphoedema may not develop. They do, however, warrant a consultation with a health professional who is knowledgeable about the diagnosis and treatment of lymphoedema, or with a breast-care or other specialist nurse. Early intervention at this stage is important and can have a significant impact on the course of lymphoedema.

Complicating factors

There are a number of factors that can increase the risk of developing lymphoedema or make an existing condition worse and harder to treat.

Matters over which we have no control include age and the onset of a disease such as cancer which requires treatment. In that event, as outlined earlier, relevant factors include the extent and type of surgery, the number of lymph vessels and nodes removed, whether the wound needs to be drained (and, if so, for how long), whether the wound becomes infected, and whether or not radiotherapy is required (and, if so, the extent of coverage).

Certain risk factors can, however, be managed, such as skin condition which is discussed in detail later in this book. Two other controllable factors are body weight and the amount of lymph requiring removal.

BODY WEIGHT

This is an important risk factor. Being overweight results in a greater than normal load of fluid requiring removal by the lymphatic system. Being overweight or obese may also be related to a condition called lipoedema (see page 13). In both cases, fatty deposits in surface tissue can hinder the functioning of the lymphatic system by reducing the carrying capacity of the lymph vessels. If lymphatic vessels have been damaged or destroyed, a person who is overweight or has lipoedema may experience more severe swelling.

THE LYMPH LOAD

Another factor that can be controlled to some extent is the lymphatic load – the amount of fluid waiting to be removed from a limb or other body part. As outlined earlier, a higher than normal lymph load may result from high blood pressure, an infection, stress, or blood vessels which are not structually sound. As noted above, it may also be higher in overweight people, simply because there is more tissue from which the fluids have to be drained.

Associated changes and conditions

The development of lymphoedema is a complicated process which is not yet fully understood.

The accumulation of fluid in the tissues which may precede lymphoedema can be so subtle that no swelling is evident (this period is called the latent or hidden phase). As noted on page 18, however, symptoms such as pain, pins and needles, heaviness, tension or cramps may indicate other potentially damaging changes and a professional medical assessment is advisable.

Chronic lymphoedema is more than just an accumulation of fluids in body tissue: there are significant changes in the number and type of cells and their activity levels, changes in the levels of oxygen in the tissues, and accumulations of protein and waste products. Among the cells that may be affected are macrophages, the white blood cells whose job it is to clear away debris such as dead or dying tissue and which are therefore central to the body's immune system and the maintenance of tissue structure. If macrophages fail to function properly, there may be a build-up of fibrous material in the tissues (fibrotic induration), which further reduces the transport capacity of lymph vessels and so increases the risk of lymphoedema.

CELLULITIS

Cellulitis is an inflammation of connective tissues which results from infection caused by streptococcal bacteria. People with lymphoedema are prone to recurrent episodes of cellulitis. Erysipelas is a similar condition involving acute inflammation of the skin and subcutaneous tissues.

Cellulitis should not be confused with cellulite, which is the common term for a lumpy contour found most commonly in the female buttocks and thighs, and which can be tender. It is likely that cellulite and lipoedema are related. Cellulite usually occurs – or, at least, is of the greatest concern – in young adulthood and around middle age. It is not caused by infection and may have a genetic component.

Cellulitis is accompanied by fever. The lymphoedema site becomes red, more swollen, tender and hot, and the effect seems to penetrate to some depth. There may be a line of redness along the line of the major lymph vessels (lymphangitis) and some tenderness in the lymph nodes of the groin or armpit. Early treatment with antibiotics is essential to control the spread of bacteria, so any symptoms of cellulitis or lymphangitis should be referred to a medical practitioner as soon as possible. If you have received antibiotic treatment for this condition in the past, your health practitioner could perhaps issue a prescription which you can have filled the moment you detect the symptoms.

Treatment options

Cellulitis may recur several times a year, but in many cases each episode lasts only two to three days and may improve after a period of rest without the need for antibiotics. However, it is important to seek medical advice the moment you perceive symptoms such as those described above.

The management of lymphoedema includes preventing and treating cellulitis. *Streptococcus* bacteria do respond to low-dose antibiotics, but these should be used in conjunction with a full regime of therapy for lymphoedema and venous (of the veins) disease. Low-cost self-help measures include elevation of the affected limb, physical activity, breathing exercises and good skin care. Further approaches, though more expensive, include bandaging or compression garments, and manual lymphatic drainage. (It has been found, however, that inflammation can result when bacterial toxins and waste products are moved from one site to another, so lymphatic drainage massage should be avoided during episodes of cellulitis as it may excacerbate the condition.) These treatments are discussed in detail in Chapters 4 and 5.

Quality skin care can also help reduce the risk of cellulitis because the natural oils (sebum) secreted from sebaceous glands in healthy skin act as a barrier against bacteria. The organisms that invade the skin and cause cellulitis are present in only 10–20 per cent of the population. They do, however, have the potential to do great harm if they penetrate deeply and cause inflammation of the tissues. This may occur if they elude the body's immune system, which can be weakened by conditions such as diabetes mellitus, AIDS and alcoholism, and more personal factors such as poor skin care. Both lymphatic and cardiovascular diseases also affect the skin's ability to repair itself.

Techniques for diagnosing lymphoedema

There are both simple and very technical objective tests that can indicate changes in a limb suspected of having lymphoedema.

Generally the tests involve comparing the limb on the side where surgery or radiotherapy has taken place with the limb on the untouched side so that the extent of change can be measured. If both limbs are at risk of lymphoedema the measurements should, if possible, be compared with those obtained from people with a healthy lymphatic system; or, failing this, comparative measurements can be made as treatment progresses.

MEASUREMENTS
Measuring the volume and circumference of a limb is the most common method of assessing changes. Patients can easily do this themselves, but should first discuss the procedure with a health professional.

Limb circumference
Circumference is usually measured along the limb at 10-centimetre intervals, beginning at the longest digit (finger or toe). The measurements are best made with an ordinary tape measure held with light but constant tension. If possible, the measurements should be made at the same time of the day (ideally in the morning) and compared with those of the normal limb. Generally, if the circumferences of the normal and affected limbs differ by 2 centimetres or more, the swelling warrants attention. Comparative measurements may, however, reveal differences as great as 1–1.5 centimetres, which often simply reflects differences in musculature, the dominant arm or leg having the larger diameter. It can be useful to graph the measurements to provide a visual record of the changes over time.

Limb volume
Although circumference measurements give a good indication of alterations in the size of a limb, determining a limb's volume provides a more accurate picture of any changes that are taking place. This may be done by immersing the limb in a cylinder of water and measuring how much water is displaced, or by using

a computer to calculate the limb's volume from its circumference measurements.

A perometer is a device which can detect and measure very accurately (at over 200 positions) subtle volume changes and show which part of the limb is affected. As yet, however, very few practitioners have this technology and accurate manual circumference measurements are just as useful, although time-consuming.

IDENTIFYING CHANGES IN BODY TISSUE
Assessing resistance to compression (tonometry)
This is a non-invasive technique to assess the body tissue's resistance to compression which is applied by a small plunger. Tonometry is useful because it indicates the type of changes that are occurring in each of the lymphatic territories (see page 6), so that treatment can be targeted at these problem areas.

Tonometry detects the accumulation of fibre in tissue (which can reduce the lymphatic vessels' transport capacity) and can pick up small variations before a limb starts changing size. The process can also provide some information about fluid accumulation.

Tonometers are not yet widely used, but it is possible to mimic their effects by a gentle pinch test in the middle of each of the major lymphatic territories. A health professional with experience in treating lymphoedema can demonstrate this procedure and how to detect differences in response in the various territories. Any concerns arising from such tests should be raised with a doctor so that possible problems can be investigated.

Bio-impedance
A bio-impedance meter is a useful tool for identifying subtle changes in the fluid content of a limb and, like tonometry, can detect differences in the limb before its size changes. This device works by passing small electrical currents of different frequencies through the tissues: the various frequencies take different pathways and the resulting data is used to calculate how much fluid is outside the cells (extracellular) and how much is inside

them (intracellular) – the former alters markedly in lymphoe-demas. A bio-impedance meter also provides a limited amount of information about other aspects of body composition such as its fat content.

DETERMINING THE CAPABILITY OF THE LYMPHATIC SYSTEM

Imaging techniques can be used to assess both the structural condition of the lymphatic system and how well the system is working.

How adequate is it?

Magnetic resonance imaging (MRI) is the method that gives the most detailed information about the condition of the lymphatic system and the parts of the body it drains. Essentially, MRI provides a computer-generated cross-section through a particular area. It shows what changes have occurred, such as thickened tissue, fibre or fluid pooling, and abnormalities in lymphatic vessels and nodes. This in turn allows comparisons to be made with normal limbs.

An ultrasound scan (which uses high-frequency sound waves to create an image) can also provide useful information about the structure of the lymphatic system. The scan can reveal the extent of fibrosis (the build-up of excess fibrous tissue) in the lymphatic territories. It also indicates the condition, number and location of lymph nodes in the root of the extremities and reveals any fibrous, hardened tissues. The main drawback with this technique is that the images are often indistinct, but the technology is improving all the time.

How well is it functioning?

The best way of assessing how well the lymphatic system is working is via an image called a lymphoscintigram. First a small amount of radioactive material is injected into two places in the web space of the fingers or toes (massage and/or gentle exercise may be required to get the tracer material moving) and pictures are then taken of the limb and other regions such as the armpit, groin or abdomen. Sometimes the movement of the lymph (and thus of the tracer) is very slow, in which case testing may have to be carried out over a whole day so that a comprehensive picture can be built up.

A lymphoscintigram provides information about the major drainage pathways, and the rates at which lymph is transported and fluid accumulates. It also reveals any areas of dermal back-flow (where lymph flows in a reverse direction and eventually accumulates in the spaces between tissues). Identifying problem regions such as these can indicate where blockages may occur and allow treatment to be targeted where it is most needed.

Lymphoscintigraphy can provide very valuable information about the transport capacity of the lymphatic system, especially after surgery, radiotherapy or injury. If the transport capacity is shown to be within the normal range, there is little (if any) risk of the patient developing lymphoedema. Where transport capacity is below normal, the patient could be at risk of developing lymph-oedema and may benefit from some form of management program.

Unfortunately this very efficient diagnostic tool is not widely used, because of its high cost.

Lymph-node biopsy
This procedure is used to detect any cancer in the first (sentinel) lymph nodes that drain from a suspected cancer site. It only removes a small amount of lymphatic tissue and so theoretically reduces the risk of lymphoedema. It is thought that sentinel nodes may indicate the condition of all the nodes in a drainage pathway and there is evidence that they may be accurate indi-cators of cancer spread. As this technology is still evolving, it is advisable for both patients and health professionals to keep informed about its current status and any associated issues.

PART 2

Managing and Treating Lymphoedema

This section focuses on approaches to managing and treating lymphoedema. Chapter 3 discusses basic approaches to managing lymphoedema, including routine measures such as good skin care. Chapter 4 outlines the importance of physical activity in the management of lymphoedema, and suggests a range of special-purpose exercises. Chapter 5 examines compression therapy (by means of bandaging or compression garments), laser therapy and/or pneumatic pumps. Chapter 6 summarises the various surgical procedures and drug therapies currently available. Chapter 7 looks at the psychological and lifestyle changes that can confront and challenge not only lymphoedema patients but also their families, friends and work colleagues. Chapter 8 discusses the part that diet – and, above all, sound nutrition – can play in lymphoedema management. Chapter 9 recommends a daily foot-care regime, and considers some common problems and treatments.

THREE

Approaches to managing lymphoedema

Some people may require very little treatment for their lymphoedema. Management may simply mean avoiding activities that aggravate the swelling and taking sensible precautions such as practising good skin care and doing special exercises. Others find that this is not enough and that they benefit from therapeutic techniques such as manual lymphatic drainage or from wearing a compression garment.

This chapter focuses on living with lymphoedema and recommends some routine management practices. Specific hands-on treatments such as targeted exercises, compression therapy, surgery or medication are covered in the following chapters.

Living with lymphoedema

First of all, a qualified lymphoedema therapist should assess the patient with a view to developing an appropriate management strategy (Lymphoedema Associations often have a list of therapists see the resources section for contact details of these associations on page 105). Further medical tests may be required in order to give the clearest possible picture of the situation. Every person (and every lymphatic system) is different and each management program should reflect this, taking into account the patient's medical history and current lifestyle.

Depending on the extent of swelling, treatment might include an intensive phase of daily manual lymphatic drainage, bandaging until the swelling reduces to a certain level, followed by the use of a compression garment and exercise to keep the swelling down.

Managing lymphoedema is very much a team approach and a number of health professionals may need to be involved. Partners/carers also have a part to play, especially where treatments such as manual lymphatic drainage are concerned.

The importance of education and experience

Education is one of the keys to successful lymphoedema management. Information about how the lymphatic system works, why it may fail to work effectively and the consequences of this is given in Part 1; further sources of information data are listed at the end of the book. It is important to ask lots of questions so that you fully understand lymphoedema, the management strategies available and the factors that can affect the condition. For example, a healthy diet is beneficial whereas being overweight or exercising too much may aggravate lymphoedema. There are even seasonal considerations, because heat tends to put an extra load on the lymphatic system. Some people find that lymphoedema is easier to control in winter than in summer, and that in summer strenuous activities such as sport or gardening are best kept for the cooler parts of the day. Some common questions are answered, where relevant, throughout this chapter.

There tend to be days when lymphoedema is less severe and days when it is worse, and learning from personal experience is a valuable management tool. As every lymphatic system is different, it is important that you learn to recognise what activities and combination of activities affect your wellbeing. A person with arm lymphoedema who vacuums the house in the morning and then gardens in the afternoon may experience aches and increased swelling in that limb at night, but have no problems at all if they only do one of those tasks. In this case, simply modifying the amount they do on any one day will keep the lymphoedema under control. For someone else, inactivity may be a problem. For instance, a person with leg lymphoedema whose job involves sitting at a desk all day may find that the swelling is worse during the week than at weekends. In this case making a habit of getting up and walking around for a short time every hour at work is likely to minimise leg problems at the end of the day.

Q *I've read that heat increases the load on my lymphatic system. So is it still okay to have hot showers, or a spa or sauna?*

A Heat does tend to increase the blood flow to the surface of the skin and so can add to the lymphatic system's workload. If you prefer hot showers, observe whether they exacerbate the swelling. If so, simply reduce the water temperature or keep the affected limb out of the path of the hot water.

Whether or not you should have a spa depends on whether you can regulate the water temperature. For example, spas at public pools and gyms are usually very hot and users cannot adjust the thermostat. The temperature of home spas or spa baths, on the other hand, is determined by the temperature of the water that runs into them and the spa heater's thermostat can be altered, so it is not difficult to have a warm spa rather than a hot one.

As saunas are invariably hot, however, they are not recommended for people with lymphoedema.

Q *I've heard that carrying heavy objects can increase lymphoedema swelling. But how heavy is 'heavy'?*

A There is no scientific evidence that carrying heavy weights will either increase or trigger lymphoedema. If you build up slowly and feel no after-effects such as aches or increased swelling, it's probably safe. It is unlikely that lifting a heavy object once will produce swelling; it is more commonly caused by repetitive lifting. But it is best to avoid lifting heavy weights you are not used to, not least because straining a muscle is likely to increase the lymph load in that region as the body repairs itself. If you must move something heavy, try to find another way of shifting the load, e.g. by dividing it up or by pushing rather than lifting it. If swelling has increased at the end of the day, think back over what you have done and try to work out which activity might have led to this change.

General tips

ARM LYMPHOEDEMA

- It is a good idea to wear gloves when using detergents (kitchen and laundry); the pH of detergents is between 7–11 (see 'Skin Care' on page 33).
- Women may find it more comfortable to wear a bra with wide straps and a wide section under the arms; a shoulder pad under the strap may also help. A bra should not be too tight across the back and extending the back strap with a hook-on section (available from large lingerie stores) may assist lymph flow to other areas.
- Avoid tight clothes and jewellery which tend to leave deep furrows in the skin when removed, as they may reduce the flow of lymph from the affected area. You may need to enlarge watchband(s), rings and other jewellery.
- It is not advisable to carry something heavy in your hand or bear heavy weight through your shoulder (e.g. a tote bag) on the lymphoedema-affected side for an extended period of time. This causes the muscles involved to be constantly contracted and lymphatic flow may be reduced as a result because the normal automatic on–off tightening of muscles is necessary to assist the passage of lymph through the system.

LEG LYMPHOEDEMA

- Cut toenails very carefully to avoid nicking or tearing the skin. If this proves too difficult or there are problems such as ingrown toenails which can pierce the skin and are therefore a potential site of infection, consult a podiatrist. (See also Chapter 9.)
- As tight underwear can impede the flow of lymph, loose garments and those with no leg elastic (such as boxers) are preferable. Socks and knee high stockings with tight or

elasticised tops should also be avoided, as they can act like a tourniquet. Below-knee medical compression stockings are not a problem because they apply graduated pressure which is strongest at the ankle and least at the knee.

- Well-fitting, supportive shoes are recommended. Low-cut shoes can exacerbate foot lymphoedema because the swelling is not supported over the top of the foot; adjustable footwear with laces or velcro fastenings may be better (see page 96).

Skin care

For someone with lymphoedema, good skin care is important for two main reasons: it helps keep the skin healthy so that this huge organ continues to act as a barrier against unwanted organisms such as bacteria or allergens and thus helps prevent the lymphatic system becoming overloaded.

In healthy skin, natural oils (sebum) secreted from the sebaceous glands keep the skin soft and supple. They also inhibit the growth of bacteria and fungi by maintaining the skin's natural acidity (bacteria and fungi prefer an alkaline environment, i.e. a pH level greater than 7).

A person with lymphoedema, or at risk of developing it, is prone to dry and undernourished skin. The skin may therefore no longer function as a protective barrier because dry skin often cracks and so provides an entry point for germs. Good skin care can help reduce the risk of developing cellulitis.

THROW AWAY THE SOAP

Soap has very undesirable effects on the skin, stripping away its protective layer of sebum and, being alkaline, destroying its natural acidity. The skin then becomes susceptible to dryness, damage, irritation and infection. Normal, healthy skin can overcome these problems fairly readily, but skin that is under stress due to swelling may take longer to recover and the lymphoedema may worsen.

When you wash your hands with soap, your skin's pH (acid–alkali) balance changes from its usual level (5.5–6.5, acidic) to a higher one (9–10, alkaline). Usually the acidic sebum secreted by the skin changes the pH back to normal in about 15 minutes, but if skin is dry or unhealthy this process can take much longer, up to two hours. If the skin is damaged during that time, the deeper layers are susceptible to invasion by bacteria and/or fungi. Many leading soap brands have a pH level of 10–12, so if you wish to use a cleansing bar, buy a soap-free formula (available from pharmacists).

Furthermore, nearly all soaps contain caustic soda, which is an irritant, especially for already damaged skin. Most soaps also contain strong perfume or other additives, which can cause problems for sensitive skin.

MOISTURISE

The main aim of moisturising creams, lotions and oils is to replace the skin's lost sebum, adding a fine greasy film which both brings moisture to the skin and reduces the amount lost through it. The emollients (softening agents) in these products also have a lubricating effect and make the skin feel smoother.

A small percentage of the population is allergic to lanolin, so lanolin-free moisturisers are recommended. As with soaps, it is best to use moisturisers that are perfume-free, because additives can aggravate any existing skin conditions. The instructions accompanying most brands of compression garment suggest avoiding moisturisers that contain vitamin E or petroleum products, not because they are harmful to skin but rather because they tend to clog up fibres and so reduce the garment's useful life.

Moisturisers should be applied to already moist skin, as this allows them to penetrate more deeply. If the skin is very dry, it may be necessary to apply these products twice a day (morning and night) and, if this isn't enough, to combine them with a perfume-free bath or shower oil or gel. If a lotion has been applied and the skin is still dry, a cream may work better. Similarly, if one brand of moisturiser has been used for a period of time and the skin remains dry, it may help to change brands.

There are a number of good products designed for dry skin, which are available from most pharmacists. But if the problem does not improve with a simple moisturising regime, consult a health professional.

PROTECT SKIN FROM THE SUN

There are many good reasons to avoid getting sunburnt, the most obvious one is to reduce the risk of skin cancer. If you do get sunburnt your body has to repair this area as well as try to reverse the temperature increase that occurs during and after exposure to the sun. The body achieves this by directing the blood to the small blood vessels close to the surface of the skin, which increases the amount of fluid and protein in the tissue spaces and so produces a greater load for the lymphatic system to remove. For someone with lymphoedema this can further overload an already compromised system; for someone at risk of developing it (after having had lymph glands removed, for example), the increased lymph load may tip the balance in a system that was previously working well. The best approach is to cover up when out in the sun – '*Slip* on a shirt. *Slop* on sunscreen. *Slap* on a hat', as the slogan says. A number of moisturisers contain a sunscreen as well (check the label). While sunscreen protection is advisable even when compression garments are worn, some sunscreens containing a moisturiser are not suitable because they clog the garment fibres (see 'Moisturise' on page 34, and Chapter 5).

Also remember that UV rays entering a car through the windscreen or windows can cause sunburn. Long sleeves are helpful, but sunscreen should also be applied to the backs of hands before car travel. Special car sleeves with an added section covering the back of the hand are available; a therapist or health professional should be able to suggest retail outlets.

Q *I have been told that I should avoid particularly damaging the skin on my swollen arm. Is this true?*

A Yes, it is important to avoid scratching or cutting a limb which has lymphoedema because this provides a way in for germs which could lead to the recurring skin infection called cellulitis. When gardening and pruning, for example, it is a good idea to wear a long-sleeved top and pants, and gardening gloves to avoid scratches from plants. It's also wise to use an insect repellent and to apply anti-itch cream (available from pharmacists and supermarkets) if you do get bitten, to lessen the need to scratch and perhaps break the skin.

At the same time, there is no need to panic if you do get cuts or scratches. Normally it's enough to clean the area, apply an antiseptic cream and then a covering, though you can expect scratches to take longer to heal if you have lymphoedema because the healing process is slowed down. It is normal for the line of the cut to become slightly inflamed and red, but if these symptoms increase and spread it may indicate an infection, in which case you should seek medical advice as soon as possible.

Q *What is the best means of shaving my leg which has lymph-oedema?*

A The main concern when shaving is to try to avoid cutting yourself, as cuts are potential access points for germs which may give rise to infection. While an electric razor is less likely than a blade to cause nicks, if not handled properly it can abrade the skin and if not cleaned properly it may become a source of bacteria, so a blade used carefully may be just as safe. People who have had lymph glands removed from the armpit and have reduced sensation in this area should be vigilant whatever shaving method they use, or ask someone else to do the job for them.

Depilatory waxing is best avoided, as the hairs are pulled out and leave small holes which may be sites for germs to enter.

Medical procedures

While it is important for lymphoedema sufferers to avoid cuts and scratches, an occasion may arise where a medical procedure involving an incision becomes necessary, such as the removal of a skin cancer, mole or solar keratosis (sun spot). Following the procedure, check the wound regularly and consult a medical practitioner if the site becomes inflamed or red, in case there is an infection. If you have had cellulitis in the past, tell the medical practitioner this: they may prescribe antibiotics as a precautionary measure.

HAVING BLOOD PRESSURE TAKEN

There is no evidence that having a blood-pressure test on an arm that has or is at risk of developing lymphoedema will exacerbate or cause the condition. It has, however, been suggested that the pressure exerted on the arm during this procedure may cause lymph to back up and overload those vessels that are still functioning. Once again, the best solution is to use the non-affected arm for the test. If lymph nodes have been removed from both armpits, blood pressure could be measured on the leg instead.

INJECTIONS AND INTRAVENOUS DRIPS

An injection, of course, involves a break in the skin but is not generally a problem as this is a sterile procedure and therefore unlikely to cause infection. There is, however, a very small chance that germs could enter via the puncture point, so it is sensible, if possible, to have the injection in a lymphoedema-free location. If that is not feasible, the puncture point should be checked regularly and a doctor consulted if the site becomes red, hot and swollen.

Q *I have arm lymphoedema. I have been told that I should never have blood taken from that arm or an intravenous drip inserted there. But the veins in the other arm are difficult to access. What choice have I got?*

A   There is no scientific evidence that having an intravenous drip inserted or blood taken from a vein in the arm, will exacerbate your conditon (or trigger lymphoedema in someone who is at risk). However, there is anecdotal evidence of malfunctioning drips sending the fluid into surrounding tissues instead of a vein, with the result that swelling occurred. In addition, although these are sterile procedures there is a small risk of infection because they involve a break in the skin and a germ could enter during or immediately following the process. If the veins in your unaffected arm are inaccessible (which can, for example, occur during chemotherapy or when there is repeated use of the veins in one arm), discuss the problem with your doctor to determine if there is another site that would be safe to use. If there is no alternative, or in the event of an emergency, your affected arm may have to be used. Bear in mind, though, that any resulting swelling can be fairly easily managed, whereas the consequences of not having blood tested or a drip inserted could be serious.

Limb elevation

Elevating a limb encourages the slow downhill drainage of lymph and the movement of fluid through the tissues. It has a profound and immediate effect in encouraging the blood in congested veins to empty and to take the load off the lymphatic system. Ideally, the limb should be raised well above the heart (see Figures 3.1 and 3.2) to encourage the slow downwards flow. This is not always comfortable or practical, however, and any degree of elevation that can be achieved during normal activities – such as putting the legs up when watching TV or resting the arm on a raised support when travelling – is helpful.

Elevation (Figures 3.1 & 3.2) is most effective for limbs with soft, early-stage lymphoedema, as lymphoedema hardens over time and thus restricts lymph flow.

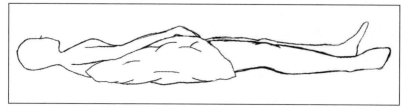

Figure 3.1 Elevation of the arm.

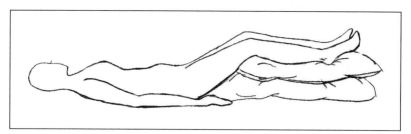

Figure 3.2 Elevation of the leg.

SLEEPING POSITIONS

It is very important for lymphoedema sufferers to have a good night's rest. If you have arm lymphoedema, you may find it beneficial to avoid sleeping on the affected side. Sleeping on your back or side with a pillow under your arm to keep it higher than your heart can assist drainage, though this can be awkward and cause broken sleep. It's best to experiment and see what works for you.

If you have leg lymphoedema, sleeping on your back with pillows under your leg(s) will assist drainage. Elevation can also be achieved by placing a firm object under the mattress or propping up the bed itself at the foot end. These positions may aggravate respiratory or gastric reflux conditions, however, so seek medical advice before you adopt this approach.

Travel tips

It pays lymphoedema sufferers to be well prepared for travelling. What to pack?

- Sunscreen, moisturiser, insect repellent and something to stop the itch (e.g. Stop Itch or vinegar) if you do get bitten.
- For hot-weather destinations, long-sleeved shirts (for arm lymphoedema) and/or lightweight trousers (for leg lymphoedema).
- A small first-aid kit, including antiseptic cream. Tea-tree oil is also a useful mild antiseptic.
- For leg lymphoedema, tinea remedies such as Tinaderm or Daktarin just in case, as this condition is commonly acquired in public conveniences and facilities. The best way to prevent tinea is to dry carefully between the toes.
- If you normally wear a compression garment, take rubber gloves and any aids you use to put the garment on, plus a small container of mild laundry detergent and a needle and thread in case minor repairs are needed. For hot-weather destinations, a small spray bottle allows the garment to be dampened with water and so keep the limb cool.
- If you have had cellulitis in the past, seek medical advice about whether it is advisable to carry antibiotics or a prescription for them. (If you are travelling overseas, it's advisable to take an explanatory letter from your doctor.)

Air travel

While there is no conclusive evidence that lymphoedema is aggravated by flying, the combination of low cabin pressure and physical inactivity, especially on long flights, may cause swelling. Booking staff should be alerted to your condition and any special needs, and again it's advisable to have a supporting letter from a medical practitioner. Even if you do not usually wear a compression garment, discuss with a therapist the advisability of wearing one during the flight. (See also page 63.)

- If you normally wear a compression garment, take two new ones with you (for optimal compression). Some people also wear an old compression garment or bandage over the new one for extra support. Consult your therapist as to the best option.
- Standard exercises can be done while seated. For long-haul flights it is also beneficial for the back as well as for lymphoedema to walk up and down the aisles every couple of hours. Consider taking a small blow-up cushion to place underfoot for exercising your legs, or a soft squeeze ball for arm exercises.
- Air travellers with arm lymphoedema should try to get a seat near a window and use the ledge to support and elevate the arm. For leg lymphoedema, a seat behind the toilet section (the bulkhead) is useful because there is generally more room to stretch out.

CAR OR BUS TRAVEL

- As for air travel, wearers of compression garments should take two new ones, though it is probably not necessary to wear two garments (or a garment plus bandage) at once.
- It is important for both the affected limb (especially if you have leg lymphoedema) and your back to stop the car every hour or so, get out and walk around. On a bus trip, take the opportunity at each stop to have a good stretch and stroll.
- If you are a passenger, practise all the exercises that are possible within the confines of your seat.

- If you are the driver and have arm lymphoedema, shift the arm around and keep things moving by gently squeezing the steering wheel. A driving sleeve may also be useful (see page 35).
- If you are a passenger, as with air travel, a small blow-up cushion for leg exercises and a soft squeeze ball for the arms are recommended.
- If you have arm lymphoedema, apply sunscreen and wear long sleeves.

Manual lymphatic drainage

As described in Chapter 1, lymph fluid drains in a particular direction depending on the area of the body affected. Lymph-oedema treatments and management approaches are generally designed either to make the lymphatic system work better and pump more lymph from the affected limb (lymphostimulatory) or to encourage new lymph vessels to grow or new pathways to form (lymphogenic).

Manual lymphatic drainage, a lymphostimulatory therapy, is a light and very slow form of massage which assists the flow of lymph along the lymphatic vessels. Many different techniques can be used, depending on which part of the body needs to be drained and how extensive the area is. The massage begins with the unaffected side of the body, then moves to the affected side and finally to the affected limb. It's a bit like unclogging a blocked pipe: just as you need to make sure the unblocked section of the pipe is flowing well before trying to clear the blockage, so manual lymphatic drainage aims first to empty the non-lymphoedema areas to create space to receive lymph from the affected region. Once the torso is clear, the limb is massaged in sections starting at the top. A therapist can teach you how to do this yourself, using a stroking technique. If appropriate, a family member or support person can also learn the techniques.

It must be stressed that other, non-specific forms of massage can exacerbate lymphoedema as they may increase the amount of fluid in the area. It is therefore essential that your massage therapist is trained in specialised lymphatic drainage techniques.

Before embarking on a course of manual lymphatic drainage, seek an assessment by a qualified lymphoedema therapist who will establish the most appropriate combination of therapies for your particular needs. In some cases, lymphatic drainage needs to be combined with the wearing of a compression garment; in other cases, it can be supplemented simply with exercises.

FOUR

The role of exercise in lymphoedema management

It is generally accepted (though not always acted upon) that regular exercise is vital for our physical and mental health. The Australian National Health and Medical Research Council (NHMRC) recommends at least thirty minutes of moderate exercise on most (preferably all) days of the week to reduce the risk of many related diseases such as heart disease, diabetes, osteoporosis, high blood pressure and obesity. What, though, is the situation for people with lymphoedema, particularly since it has been reported that intense physical activity can precipitate the condition?

The fact is that exercise has a key role to play in the management of lymphoedema. Physical activity not only helps force fluid through the lymphatic vessels but also takes some of the load off the venous system. As noted in Chapter 3, the sooner treatment commences following the diagnosis of lymphoedema, the better the outcome. During the early stage of lymphoedema, exercise, together with good skin care, can reduce symptoms and may avert the need for massage or compression garments. Physical activity also triggers the release of the 'happy' chemicals called endorphins, which are believed to have an anti-depressant action. Many people describe feeling 'high' immediately after strenuous exercise, and report feeling more relaxed, less stressed and better able to sleep when they have exercised. Another recent study has shown that patients undergoing chemotherapy were less affected by fatigue, nausea and depression if they were involved in a daily exercise program.

What sort of exercise?

Specialised exercises have been developed which encourage lymphatic flow; but exercises to improve fitness and build strength are also important for people with lymphoedema.

Where lymphoedema is concerned, moving at a natural pace, with as full a range of muscular and joint action as possible, is better than vigorous, once-daily exercise. While energetic movement to strengthen the heart and other muscles and to burn up calories is good for some medical conditions, it is not what the lymphatic and venous systems need. Slow and varied movements are enough to empty the veins without forcing fluid out of the blood vessels into the tissues, which can worsen lymphoedema. A full range of ankle movements is especially important for those with lymphoedema of the lower leg: the ankle is the stiffest and most immobile joint in such cases, and exercises are effective for emptying the venous and lymphatic systems in that part of the limb.

It is advisable to develop an exercise regime with the guidance of a lymphoedema physiotherapist. First discuss your particular needs with your physiotherapist; one person may be able to play tennis with no increase in arm swelling while another may be able to walk 10 kilometres with no worsening of their leg swelling. It is therefore important to try to determine the 'right' level of exercise for you, one which will not overload your lymphatic system: possible signs of an overloaded system are increased aching, heaviness and, of course, swelling. If you have always led a physically active life you should adapt to lymphoedema-specific exercises without difficulty. If you have never been the 'exercise type', it's a good opportunity to find out how good it feels to be fitter and more supple as well as managing your lymphoedema! Exercise should be introduced gradually so that both you and the therapist can monitor its effects constantly and modify the program accordingly. For example, someone with leg lymphoedema who wants to return to playing golf could perhaps start with a bucket of balls on the practice fairway and progress to playing a few holes before attempting nine or eighteen holes.

ENCOURAGING LYMPHATIC FLOW

As outlined in Chapter 1, lymphatic flow is brought about by the pumping action of the deeper lymphatic vessels which have smooth muscle in their walls and valves along their length. The contracting of the segments between each set of valves causes lymph to flow centrally, eventually emptying into the large veins near the heart. The flow of lymph is also assisted by body movements, the pumping action of arteries and the heart, and by regular movement of the lungs and diaphragm when breathing. Physical activity is of particular benefit because contracting muscles and moving joints compress and stretch the lymphatic system and so drive the lymph towards the heart.

Specialised exercises designed to improve lymphatic flow have been shown to reduce oedema in an affected limb. These exercises should be performed slowly (a count of five seconds for each movement, followed by a rest of equal length) and in a designated order. If you normally wear a compression garment, you should wear it while exercising and also keep the affected limb elevated if practicable.

The following is a typical sequence of exercises to improve lymph flow. The actual form of the exercises should be determined by a physiotherapist or lymphoedema practitioner.

1. Six diaphragmatic breaths (also called abdominal or tummy breathing): the abdomen should expand with each intake of breath while the ribcage and upper chest remain reasonably still. (Figure 4.1.)
2. Self-massage to the functioning lymph nodes in the armpit, groin or neck, as demonstrated by the physiotherapist.
3. Exercise of the root (top) part of the affected limb, i.e. the hip region for legs (Figure 4.2) and the neck (Figure 4.3) and shoulder region for arms (Figure 4.4).
4. Exercise of the middle area (e.g. knee or elbow) of the affected limb (Figures 4.5 and 4.6)

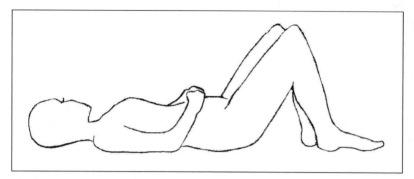

Figure 4.1 Diaphragmatic breathing.

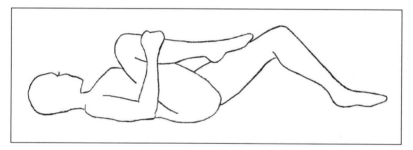

Figure 4.2 Exercise for the hip region.

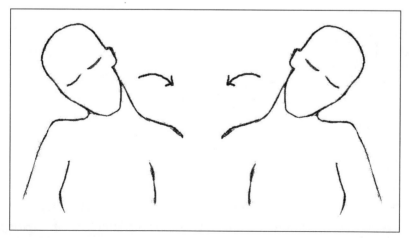

Figure 4.3 Exercise for the neck.

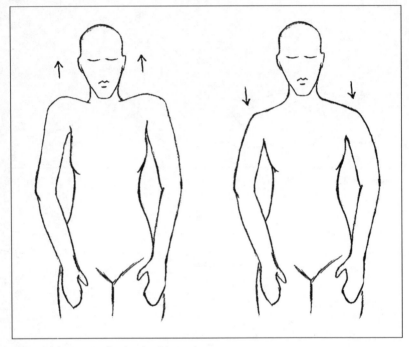

Figure 4.4 Exercise for the shoulder region.

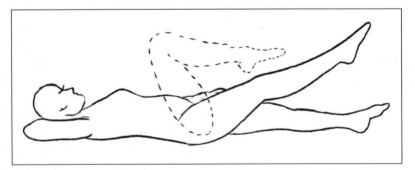

Figure 4.5 Exercise for the knee.

5. Exercise of the hand or foot (Figure 4.7).
6. Exercise involving the whole limb.

Each of the limb exercises should be repeated eight to ten times. As you become familiar with the routine, the number of repetitions can be increased.

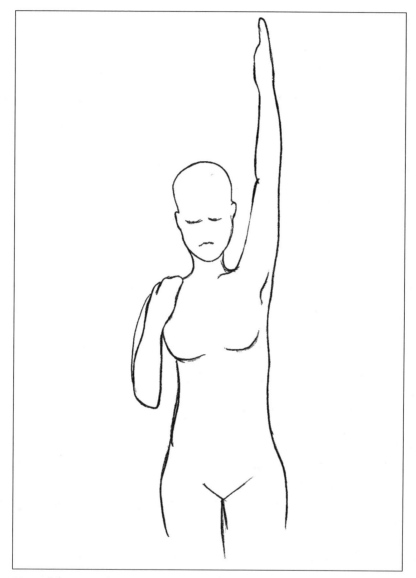

Figure 4.6 Exercise for the elbow and shoulder. Alternate raising of left and right arm.

Diaphragmatic breathing should be repeated regularly throughout the exercise session.

It is important to perform the exercises slowly, as described above, because this allows the lymph to flow smoothly and

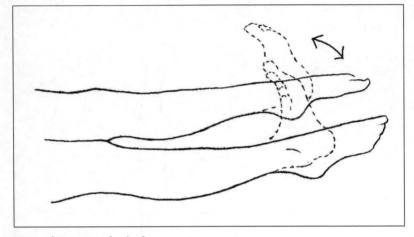

Figure 4.7 Exercise for the foot.

centrally along the lymphatic channels and will not stress the system.

IMPROVING FITNESS

This type of exercise is familiar to us all – an aerobic workout, the sort which makes us huff and puff and has long been recognised as an important strategy for the prevention and management of age-related diseases such as diabetes, hypertension, heart disease and osteoporosis.

Brisk walking, jogging, swimming, cycling, cross-country skiing, rowing, aerobic routines (including aqua aerobics) and in-line skating are all forms of aerobic exercise. (Even a good session of gardening, housework or home maintenance will do on some days.) The best form of exercise is the one that you enjoy most and is easiest to do on a regular basis; some people prefer to join a club, others to exercise with a friend or even alone. And when the weather does not suit outdoor activities, there's always the local recreation centre or gym with pool, exercise bikes, treadmills and other equipment. Aerobic exercise really is a great tonic, as anyone will agree who has discovered the benefits of a healthier and fitter body.

BUILDING STRENGTH

Strength (or resistance) training involves lifting a load in a controlled, repetitive manner to strengthen muscles and reduce muscle loss. As the muscle strengthens over time, the load is gradually increased until an optimal level is achieved which will ensure ongoing benefits.

Muscle strength decreases by 30–40 per cent during adulthood. As muscle mass decreases, the metabolic rate slows, appetite declines, energy levels reduce, the body continues to weaken and there is an increased risk of falls, injury and fractures. In some cases, nutritional problems may also result. Women are even more vulnerable than men to muscle changes with increasing age.

Strength training has only recently been recognised as having particular health and fitness benefits for the middle-aged and elderly. A 1990 study into the advantages of strength training involved people from a centre for the frail aged in Boston, USA: all the subjects were over 90 years of age, whereas all previous research had involved people under 80 who were still healthy and living in the community. The study found that high-intensity weight training can produce dramatic increases in muscle strength, even in the very frail aged.

Resistance training should focus primarily on the main muscle groups that are important for everyday activities, such as those in the shoulders, upper arms, spine, hips, thighs and calves. Exercises recommended for people with lymphoedema include biceps curls, overhead arm presses, standing up from a chair and slowly lowering again without using the hands to push off (Figure 4.8), and calf raises (Figure 4.9) – all of which can be performed with minimal equipment in the comfort of your home.

If done as described, strength training exercises will also improve lymphatic flow. They should be performed slowly, done regularly if possible (e.g. three 20-minute sessions a week), and with a bandage or compression garment (if applicable) securely in place. The resistance or weight should initially be relatively light so that the muscles are not overtaxed, and then be increased

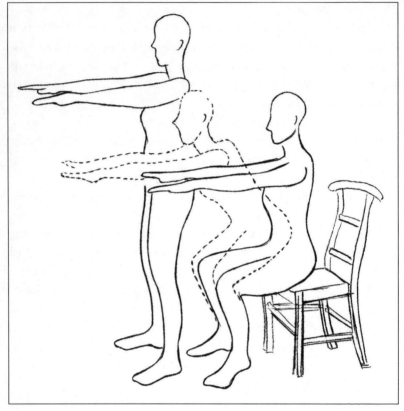

Figure 4.8 Standing up from a chair and slowly lowering.

only gradually. Some exercises use only the body as the resistance weight, such as rising onto tiptoes, and standing up from and sitting down in a chair.

If you prefer company when you exercise you could use the local gym, with a program designed by the fitness instructor. Alternatively, a physiotherapist could design and monitor a home-based program or suggest a community-based one. If you are ever unsure about any aspect of your program, contact your physiotherapist or trainer.

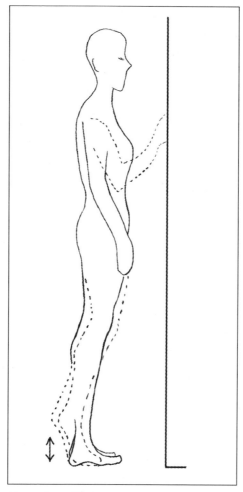

Figure 4.9 Calf raises.

Some general exercise tips

- If you have not done any exercise for some time, seek a doctor's opinion before commencing.
- If the form of exercise you do puts any strain on the lymph-oedema site (e.g. the wrist and forearm area when playing tennis), begin gradually and have some way of objectively measuring the limb to determine how the exercise affects it.

This may be as simple as measuring the wrist or taking note of the tightness of rings.

- Wear comfortable and loose-fitting clothes, with no constricting elastic or bands.
- Compression garments are not generally required for swimming or aqua aerobics because the pressure exerted on a limb when it is submerged will be sufficient, but it is sensible to consult a lymphoedema practitioner. The greater the water depth, the more pressure is exerted on the limb and therefore the greater the effect on the whole circulatory system. Lymph flow is enhanced by exercising gently in water up to, but not exceeding, 34°C, though a cooler pool is preferable for lap swimming.
- For outdoor exercise, use adequate sunscreen and insect repellent, re-applying as recommended. Exercise should be avoided during the hottest part of the day, because this could exacerbate the swelling.
- It is important to warm up and stretch before embarking on any exercise, and to cool down afterwards. This may be as simple as beginning at a slow pace and gradually getting faster, then slowing down again towards the end of the session.
- The duration and intensity of the exercise can be gradually increased, although the lymphoedema should be monitored carefully in case it flares up.
- Drinking plenty of water is essential, particularly if exercising over a longer period or in warm weather.

FIVE

Compression therapy, laser therapy and compression pumps

This chapter considers various forms of treatment using aids designed to reduce lymphoedema swelling.

As its name suggests, *compression therapy* involves applying pressure to a limb with lymphoedema so as to control or reduce the swelling. This is most commonly achieved by multi-layer bandaging or by specialised garments such as sleeves or stockings. *Laser therapy* involves passing laser beams over hardened tissue caused by flawed lymphatic drainage. A *compression pump* works by pushing fluid from the affected limb towards the trunk (torso) and so helps reduce swelling. Pumps should only be used in combination with other treatments, and only under professional supervision.

Compression therapy

For many people, compression therapy is an essential tool in the management of lymphoedema. It can maintain and enhance the results achieved by manual lymphatic drainage and keep swelling down over the long term. Compression therapy is also used to treat a range of other conditions such as burns and scars, leg ulcers and vein disorders.

The amount of pressure needed to maintain or reduce a swollen limb is an individual matter. Usually, more severe lymphoedema requires greater compression and legs usually require greater compression than arms due to the effects of gravity.

Compression therapy aids fluid movement in the limb by:

- improving the flow of blood and lymph by supporting the vessels and tissues in the limb;
- providing a firm surface for muscles to work against (exercise is most effective when done while wearing compression garments or bandages);
- softening thickened, hard (fibrose) tissues;
- conserving the benefits obtained with lymphatic drainage massage; and
- maintaining and improving the shape of the limb.

Compression of a limb should apply most pressure on the hand or foot, easing off further up the limb to allow fluid to drain away.

When compression therapy is not appropriate

Compression therapy is not suitable for everyone and the therapist must consider the complete picture before prescribing a compression garment. Special care needs to be taken in the following situations, before compression therapy is applied:

- *Poor blood flow through the arteries.* This can be caused by some medical conditions, such as diabetes. Blood flow may need to be tested before compression is applied; this is a quick and painless procedure.
- *Poor sensation in the limb.* If any areas are numb or have reduced feeling, special care is needed when wearing a compression garment and affected areas should be checked regularly to ensure the garment is not abrading the skin.
- *The presence of infection.* A compression garment should not be worn in the event of acute cellulitis (see page 20). The doctor or therapist should be consulted before the garment is worn again, which is usually when antibiotic treatment has commenced.
- *Radiotherapy.* During and immediately after radiotherapy, the skin in the area being treated can be fragile and sensitive.

Pulling a compression garment on and off may rub the skin, so the advisability of compression therapy during treatment should be discussed with a lymphoedema practitioner.

- *Fragile or sensitive skin.* Special care is needed with compression garments if the skin is prone to blistering or ulceration. (See 'Ensuring a correct fit' on page 62.)

Types of compression therapy

Compression can be applied by bandaging or by a specialised garment. A person with mild lymphoedema may be able to be fitted with a compression garment straight away, which may help maintain or slightly reduce the swelling. Someone with more severe swelling, or a limb that fluctuates in size, may need to have the limb reduced and stabilised with a program of manual lymphatic drainage and compression bandaging. It is essential to wear compression garments to maintain any reduction in swelling achieved by bandaging.

COMPRESSION BANDAGING

Bandaging is usually done for short periods of time only. It is useful for people who have extremely fragile skin or wounds, because the bandages will not stress the skin as they are put on and off. Multi-layer bandaging is also the most appropriate form of compression for reducing limbs that are particularly large or hard; bandages conform to the limb as it reduces, whereas a garment may become loose and therefore ineffectual.

Bandaging does have some disadvantages:

- Thick bandages can be bulky to wear and limit movement and lifestyle.
- You should not drive a car when wearing thick bandaging, as movement may be restricted.
- Replacing the bandages daily is time-consuming and requires daily visits to a therapist.

COMPRESSION GARMENTS

Compression garments are more practical than bandages for long-term wear. They are made of an elastic fabric that fits closely to the limb, so normal clothes can be worn on top. In addition, they are available in a range of styles and colours, and most people find them much more acceptable to wear than bandages.

It is a good idea to have two garments: this allows one to be washed while the other is being worn, and prolongs the life of both garments by allowing the elastic to 'rest'.

Selecting compression garments

There are many different types and styles of compression garments, and there are a number of issues for the therapist and wearer to consider which will determine what type of garment is most appropriate. These include the severity of the lymphoedema, the shape and size of the limb, physical capabilities (such as hand strength, ability to reach the feet, ability to take the garment off) and the condition and sensitivity of the skin. Also important, of course, are lifestyle, occupation and personal taste: a garment is no use sitting in a drawer!

READY-MADE GARMENTS

A large range of ready-made garments is available from the different specialist companies (a therapist can advise). The garments come in various styles, fabrics and colours, and also vary in the amount of pressure they provide; most can be modified. Ready-made garments are designed to fit limbs of reasonably standard shape and dimensions.

Ready-made arm sleeves are available either with gloves attached or finishing at the wrist. They may be held in place by a strap across the body or, for women, by attaching them to the bra strap (Figure 5.1). Compression gloves are available with long or short fingers, or simply as a gauntlet with a thumbpiece only.

For the legs, there are below-the-knee socks, thigh-length

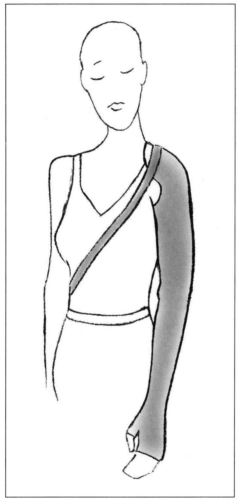

Figure 5.1 An example of an arm and hand compression garment.

stockings (some versions attach at the waist), or pantyhose (Figure 5.2).

CUSTOM-MADE GARMENTS

Compression garments can be tailor-made if a non-standard style or amount of compression is required, or if the wearer has other

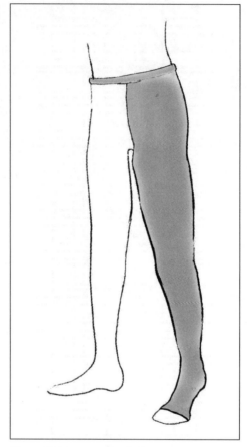

Figure 5.2 An example of a leg compression garment.

special needs. Custom-made garments are usually more expensive than ready-made ones and can take longer to obtain.

Guidelines for wearing compression garments

Exactly when a compression garment is needed will vary according to the severity of the swelling, and to lifestyle and other individual factors. This should be planned with the therapist who is prescribing the garments.

Compression garments are essential after any course of lymphatic drainage massage and compression bandaging. They may need to be worn day and night until the limb stabilises, but thereafter (in consultation with the therapist) can usually be worn during the daytime only.

Any garment that is loose, stretched or worn through needs to be replaced. Compression garments should be replaced regularly (every four to six months), because they gradually lose their elasticity and effectiveness.

GETTING GARMENTS ON AND OFF

Compression garments must fit firmly in order to do their job. This can make putting them on and taking them off quite difficult, which can be discouraging. It is a good idea to experiment with different techniques to find one that suits. Some people find it easier to turn the foot or hand section of the garment inside out, put the garment onto their hand or foot and then pull it up over the rest of the limb. Others gradually ease the garment on, smoothing it up over the limb and positioning the hand or foot last.

Several manufacturers also produce equipment to help get compression garments on and off. These include frames which hold garments open while the hand or foot is placed inside; these are helpful for people who cannot reach their feet. Other aids are designed to reduce friction, providing a slippery surface which makes it easier to draw the garment on. Aids vary in terms of how they work, how difficult they are to use, and their cost. It is advisable to discuss the options with a therapist.

Following are some simple tips for getting garments on and off. As some compression garments are inclined to slip down with movement and gravity, there are also some suggestions for keeping them in place:

- Rubber gloves are essential for gripping the fabric to ease the garment up and down. This minimises snagging, over-stretching and ripping.

- The garment should be put on early in the morning, when the limb is at its smallest.
- Compression garments tend to grab moist skin. Having a shower and moisturising the skin at night rather than in the morning will help ensure that the skin is dry by the time the garment is put on. A dusting of talcum powder can also help.
- A plastic bag or pouch of slippery fabric on the foot or hand may help a garment slip on more easily; the bag or pouch can then be pulled out through the toe or wrist hole.
- Body glue (available from therapists) or suspenders may help hold garments up.
- Bicycle shorts or a loose-fitting panty girdle can help keep stockings in place, but should not be so tight that they obstruct lymphatic flow.
- Shoulder pads can minimise the discomfort caused by the compression garment bunching behind the knee or ankle.
- Flexible adhesive dressings such as Fixomull or Hypafix (available from pharmacists) may stop a new garment rubbing in the elbow crease or behind the knee.

ENSURING A CORRECT FIT

It is essential that a compression garment fits well. Comfort is also important, of course, and some ways to ensure fit and comfort are suggested below.

- Make sure that the fabric is evenly spread along the limb, which ensures that the pressure is correctly distributed.
- Do not roll or fold down the garment top; if there is excess fabric at the top, ease the garment down over the length of the limb to ensure the fabric is evenly distributed.
- Make sure there are no creases or wrinkles, as these act like elastic bands and impede lymphatic flow.
- Garments should feel very firm and supportive, but should not be painful to wear or cause fingers or toes to turn purple or blue. If the limb aches after a period of inactivity, there may be a build-up of fluid; moving around and exercising the limb may help.

If you have any concerns about how a garment fits, take these up with the prescribing therapist.

CARE OF GARMENTS

- Always follow the manufacturer's instructions.
- Hand-wash garment in lukewarm water with mild detergent (do not machine-wash). Squeeze out excess water in a towel and dry garment in the shade. Do not tumble-dry or use direct heat.
- Avoid petroleum-based creams or lotions because these can cause the elastic in the material to deteriorate.

A NOTE FOR AIR TRAVELLERS

The jury is still out as to the best way to manage travel and lymphoedema. Some people have reported increased swelling during or shortly after travel. While many therapists believe compression may be useful, to date there is no conclusive research that proves whether or not compression while travelling can prevent swelling. The additional swelling may be due to the trip itself, or to other factors such as being extra-active when preparing for the journey, carrying heavy baggage, or giving up exercise and management regimes while on holiday.

Until further evidence is available, it seems sensible to take any simple precautions that will minimise potential problems and worry. Anyone who has a compression garment is advised to wear it; for others it is a personal decision whether or not to purchase one for the trip. Discuss this with your therapist or doctor.

Even a garment worn only occasionally for travel must be well-fitting (see page 62). If a compression garment does not fit well, or digs into the limb at the elbow or knee during periods of sitting it may exacerbate the swelling.

Laser therapy

This form of treatment involves passing laser beams over hardened lymphoedema-affected tissue. It uses a gentle form of laser (helium neon and gallium arsenide) which essentially delivers high-intensity light beams and only a low level of energy. There are two approaches: scanning, where a laser beam is moved over a site up to 10 × 20 centimetres in area; and a spot laser, used over a surgical or radiotherapy scar.

Laser therapy has been used for more than 2000 patients in South Australia at the Flinders Medical Center's Lymphoedema Assessment Clinic and Laser and Lymphoedema Clinic. 'Spot' therapy is currently being further trialled in a number of centres. So far, results suggest that laser treatment – used alone or in conjunction with other therapies such as massage – significantly reduces the amount of hardened tissue and fluid outside the cells, and the size of swollen limbs. Just as importantly, patients have reported significantly decreased discomfort, heaviness and tension in the affected limb.

Laser treatment is not a miracle cure, however. It works best for patients with considerable hardening of the tissue in one or more lymphatic territories, or in other sites where lymphatic drainage is flawed.

Compression pumps

A compression pump works by pushing fluid from the affected limb towards and partly into the trunk (torso) and so helps reduce swelling. Prior to the introduction of complex physical therapy (see Chapter 3), pneumatic devices (commonly called pumps) were frequently used as a method of treatment for lymphoedema (Figure 5.3). Experts now generally agree, however, that a pump should only ever be used in conjunction with other treatments and only under professional supervision. As with complex physical therapy, the reduction achieved with a pump needs to be maintained with compression bandages and/or a sleeve/stocking.

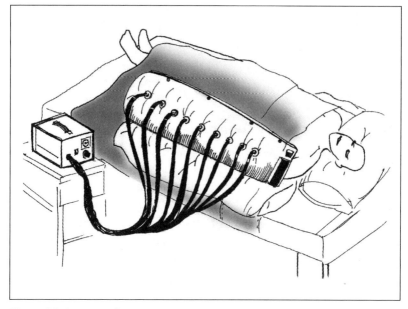

Figure 5.3 One type of compression pump.

A BRIEF HISTORY

The first pumps consisted of an inflatable plastic sleeve which encased the affected limb (including the hand or foot). The limb was then elevated and a small compressor inflated the sleeve, with the parameters (pressure, length of compression, rest periods) being set individually. There was invariably a small reduction in the swelling and it was often found that the limb had softened. After the treatment, a single layer of elastic tubular bandage would be applied to maintain the reduction. Patients received treatment twice weekly, but the reduction in swelling was often lost between sessions and the treatment was discontinued after a short time.

This single-chamber pump was later developed into a sequential compression device, in which multiple chambers inflate in sequence from the distal (furthest, i.e. hand or foot) end to the proximal (top, i.e. shoulder or hip) area, in a set cycle but with variable compression. The pump proved very popular because it could be applied without a physiotherapist in constant attendance and was particularly well received in rural areas, where few trained therapists were available. The pump could be put on and the 'work' be done while the patient watched TV or read a book. This resulted in a very passive, rather than proactive, approach to the management of lymphoedema.

THE PROS AND CONS OF COMPRESSION PUMPS

This section summarises the published findings of experts in Europe and Australia on the use of compression pumps. For more detailed information, see References section on page 101.

Lymphoedema affects not only the limb but also the adjacent part of the trunk or the area closest to the limb. Using a pump to push more fluid into an already overloaded system is likely to create even greater problems. For this reason, before a pump is applied the trunk should be prepared by manual lymphatic drainage to create a reservoir for the fluid arriving from the limb. As the limb also needs attention, you or your therapist should stroke the area above the sleeve while the pump is applied, to enhance lymph flow towards the trunk; frequent self-massage of the lymph nodes, trunk and top of the limb every 5–10 minutes is also recommended.

If this massage is not done, the following problems may result:

- The pump will push the protein-rich fluid up to the end of the sleeve, where it will accumulate and form a fibrous band. This will further hinder the flow of lymph away from the affected site. Some fluid may move into the trunk, but the protein will stay in the limb and may cause unwanted pathological changes.
- There may be increased oedema above the sleeve. In the case of leg lymphoedema, the fluid is pushed towards the hip but may also be pushed sideways into the genital area. An American study of leg lymphoedema accompanied by genital swelling found that the group treated with a pump had a 43 per cent higher incidence of genital lymphoedema than the control group.
- Some fluid might be pushed in the direction of the fingers or

toes rather than towards the body. It is therefore advisable to bandage the fingers or toes as a preventive measure, especially if the hand or foot is very swollen.

SUMMARY OF RECOMMENDATIONS

- A pump should never be used as the sole form of treatment.
- Use of a pump should always be supervised by a therapist.
- It is very important to prepare the trunk, as described above, before applying a pump. It is equally important to treat the top end of the limb during and after using a pump.
- A pump is not recommended where there is primary leg lymphoedema. Its use should, in fact, be considered carefully for any leg lymphoedema because of the risk of genital swelling.
- The maximum recommended pressure for both pump and manual lymphatic drainage is 45 mmHg.
- The reduced swelling achieved with a pump needs to be maintained with a compression garment.

SIX

Surgery and drug therapy

Lymphoedema is remarkable for the extent to which its onset, course and response to treatment varies between individuals. This, combined with the fact that variations can occur from day to day, makes it difficult to accurately assess the effects of treatment and formulate recommendations.

It is clear, however, that current surgical options offer potential benefits to selected patients, particularly those whose lymphoedema is resistant to massage, compression and exercise therapy. On the other hand, side effects limit the use of drug therapy.

New technologies such as tissue engineering and the prefabrication of blood and lymph vessels through in-vitro and in-vivo techniques are exciting new developments which may provide further treatment options in the future.

Surgery

Many surgical techniques have been assessed in trials, but this chapter only discusses those which are currently in use.

Broadly, lymphoedema surgery is used either to debulk a swollen limb or to restore the drainage pathways. Reconstruction of blocked lymphatic pathways is designed to bypass the obstruction and divert lymph flow into the venous system. Surgical intervention does not, however, offer a complete cure, and patients and doctors who understand its limitations are more likely to be satisfied with the results.

Debulking procedures

This form of surgery can immediately and significantly reduce the size of a swollen limb and bring great relief to the patient. Such procedures do not address the underlying cause of the lymph-oedema and so the condition commonly recurs unless compression garments are worn. Debulking is most effective for the upper part of the limb but does not improve lymphoedema of the hand or foot – which may, in fact, be aggravated, particularly if the surgery is extensive.

Debulking procedures, which are outlined below, range from the minimally invasive to the radical.

LIPOSUCTION

Liposuction to debulk a swollen limb involves vacuuming out lymphoedema-affected fatty tissue via thin metal 'straws' inserted into the skin. The benefit of liposuction is that it produces few side effects and little scarring, and does not appear to affect the limb's residual lymphatic function. Liposuction can be used in conjunction with other procedures, or repeated.

Liposuction plus ongoing compression therapy has been shown to reduce arm swelling by 106 per cent over a year, effectively reducing the arm to a normal size. There was a recurrence of swelling in the long term, but not to the original level. A reduced incidence of cellulitis has also been reported.

Using liposuction in conjunction with compression therapy seems to reduce swelling more than compression alone can achieve. At the same time, compression therapy is necessary to keep the swelling down. In other words, liposuction is a useful adjunct rather than a stand-alone solution; when used in isolation it achieves only about an 18 per cent reduction in volume and the swelling builds up again over time.

DEFATTING AND LIMITED EXCISION

This involves surgical defatting of lymphoedematous tissue or excising a wedge that includes both skin and underlying tissue. These procedures result in significant scarring and there may be problems with wound-healing, so they are best reserved for very swollen limbs that are resistant to other forms of treatment.

Combining limited defatting with lymphatic reconstruction maximises the benefits of both techniques.

RADICAL EXCISION

This is the most radical of the surgical procedures. It involves cutting out the affected skin and soft tissue to the level of the underlying muscle, followed by a skin graft. Obviously this is an extensive procedure and it does leave the limb disfigured. Nevertheless, it offers dramatic relief of symptoms and improved appearance in very advanced cases of lymphoedema where the limb can be quite misshapen and have very limited function as a result, and where there may even be some leakage of lymph fluid through the skin.

Lymphatic reconstruction

This procedure is suitable where the lymphatic system is blocked but otherwise likely to be functioning normally, as with someone who develops secondary lymphoedema following injury to the upper part of the limb or surgery and/or radiotherapy to the lymphatic tissue of the groin or axilla (armpit). Successful reconstruction of the lymphatic pathway is likely to have lasting benefits. Patients with primary lymphoedema that has developed spontaneously and without obvious cause are not suitable candidates.

BYPASS MICROSURGERY

The development of microsurgery made possible trialling of the procedure known as lymphovenous anastomosis (bypassing an obstruction by joining lymphatic vessels to a nearby vein). The joins can be made at various locations in the limb, though it is preferable to target the uppermost part of the limb so that as much of it as possible is drained. The procedure only requires small skin incisions and these heal rapidly. The trial results, published in the *British Journal of Plastic Surgery* (refer page 102), recorded lasting benefits in 40 per cent of patients, many of whom had no need for support measures such as massage, exercise and compression. The limb lost around 40 per cent of the excess swelling, which left it still swollen but improved the patient's self-image and quality of life. Importantly, in these patients the common skin infection cellulitis occurred less often than it had before the procedure. A further 20 per cent of patients remained static, while in the remaining 40 per cent their lymphoedema continued to develop. While the results suggest only moderate benefits, these were achieved with relatively few side effects. Limb elevation and compression therapy are required before and after this procedure, which can also be combined with debulking.

LYMPHATIC GRAFTING

This also involves bypassing a lymphatic obstruction, but the affected vessels are joined to a normal lymphatic vessel or vein which is then joined to another vessel above the obstruction. This keeps the lymphatics open and incorporates in the system a vein with one-way valves that direct flow away from the affected limb. Obtaining a normal lymphatic vessel involves an extensive incision in the other limb, however, and this is the less preferred option.

LYMPH NODE TRANSPLANTS

This involves microsurgery to transplant normal lymph nodes into a limb with lymphoedema, providing a bridge and so helping restore lymphatic flow. It is potentially of particular benefit for lymphoedema of the lower limb.

While still at a relatively experimental stage, it is thought that this procedure may in future have wider application and offer improved outcomes in selected patients.

Drug therapy

Today, medication is generally used to treat lymphoedema complications rather than the condition itself. Antibiotics, for example, are used in the treatment of cellulitis, sometimes as a long-term preventive measure.

SEVEN

Psychological and lifestyle considerations

The challenge of managing lymphoedema extends well beyond the physical. It impacts on patients' psychological and social wellbeing and that of family, friends and work colleagues. This chapter explores some of the common reactions to lymphoedema diagnosis and suggests a number of coping strategies.

It is important for lymphoedema patients to know that other people have similar feelings and that they are not alone in their responses. At the same time, each person's reaction is individual, as is the way they deal with the situation. Your emotional responses are likely to fluctuate: there will be 'good' days when you manage well, and days when you find it difficult to cope. Whatever the reaction, it is crucial to know that you have some control over your feelings. The keys to this include maintaining a positive outlook and making use of the support systems available.

Why me?

Lymphoedema may occur without warning or it may develop over a period of time. It can be triggered by something specific, such as an injury, or it can happen for no apparent reason. This unpredictability means that its onset is likely to elicit many different reactions, but perhaps the most common one is frustration. A tardy diagnosis, for example, can be upsetting, especially when little medical support has been forthcoming ('It's only a mild case of swelling. You'll have to learn to live with it'). This may in turn lead to feelings of despair and helplessness, and sometimes anger.

For people with primary lymphoedema, the road to diagnosis can be a long one. Being overweight can confuse the issue. You may have to consult several health professionals before lymphoedema is even mentioned or a correct diagnosis is made. Persisting in obtaining a diagnosis can take both courage and resourcefulness. When the condition is finally identified and steps are taken to begin appropriate treatment, you may feel a real sense of relief.

The scenario can be quite different for those who develop lymphoedema after treatment for cancer or after a trauma to the lymphatic system. Initially, it may be feared that the swelling is connected with the cancer. Even when that fear is allayed, knowing the real cause can be profoundly disappointing and sometimes depressing. Someone who has already faced a life-threatening illness is likely to wonder 'Why does this have to happen to me?'. The lymphoedema may occur just when life is beginning to return to some degree of normality: it's like a cruel reminder of what you have been through. Feelings of frustration are common too, because just as it seems possible to resume activities that had to be put on hold, the swelling produces a setback.

Lifestyle changes

A lymphoedema diagnosis can bring about a great sense of loss – loss of the capacity to do things that are important to you.

When lymphoedema interferes with work, leisure and everyday activities, the loss is acutely felt. You may feel that your independence is threatened because you cannot carry out the tasks you expect to be able to do. This has implications for friends, family and work colleagues. It can be important to reassess priorities at this time and confirm that you have much to offer in spite of that incapacity. To do so, it is often necessary to acknowledge the loss and allow yourself time to grieve before it is possible to move forward.

TAKING CONTROL

It is common for people with lymphoedema to feel that they have lost control of their life, that the swelling dictates what they can and cannot do. It is important to recognise that you can take control and that there are significant ways in which you can look after yourself and make a difference. Rather than focusing on the frustration, energy can be directed towards self-care.

The main goal is to manage the swelling effectively so that it does not dominate your life. Understanding lymphoedema and its treatment helps allay frustration and distress, so it is important to seek as much information as possible about the condition and to establish a good professional support network. On a practical level, just doing things a little differently can lessen everyday frustrations. Large jobs like weeding the garden are better divided up to make the task more manageable. Adapting to change takes time.

Sharing the burden

People need support to manage lymphoedema effectively. As with any illness, it is essential that those close to you are given the opportunity to understand the condition and what it involves. It is therefore productive to sit down with family and friends and talk about ways you might achieve your goals. Involving family and friends in some aspects of managing lymphoedema – massage, for example – is not only helpful but also lets the helper feel useful. Many people have established a closer, more intimate relationship as a result of massage, which is a shared experience from which both of you can benefit.

BUILDING SELF-ESTEEM AND CONFIDENCE

Self-esteem and confidence are probably the most important attributes for emotional stability. Self-esteem means recognising that you are valued – by yourself and by the people who are important to you. It may take some work to improve your self-esteem, especially when an experience like lymphoedema threatens your confidence.

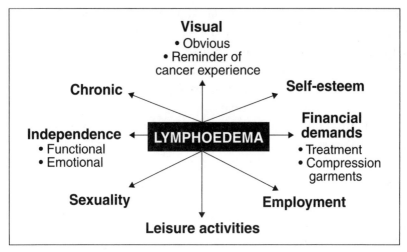

Figure 7.1 Lymphoedema can have unwanted impact on a number of areas of a person's lifestyle.

The following are a few ways to improve self-esteem:

- Be assertive. Speak up for yourself, ask for what you want and express your feelings, preferences and opinions openly and without fear.
- Keep your thoughts focused in the present, rather than living in the past or future.
- Treat yourself lovingly at every opportunity.
- Positively acknowledge yourself frequently and keep a mental note of your past achievements and accomplishments.
- Accept the acknowledgements and compliments of others. Say 'thank you' and enjoy the praise without embarrassment.
- Be respectful of the feelings and opinions of other people.

DEALING WITH OTHER PEOPLE'S REACTIONS

A positive self-image helps us deal more effectively with the reactions of others, whether they are positive or negative. You are less likely to receive negative comments or glances when you feel confident, happy and assured.

So, be prepared. A woman with lymphoedema of her right leg said: 'When I meet people, I always have to decide at what time

I am going to tell them why one leg is three times as big as the other. Otherwise, they will wonder until the time they feel it is all right to ask. I usually get in first.' Being ready with an appropriate response is a good way to keep control of a conversation or situation. It is important to answer firmly, comically or truthfully, depending on the situation.

Usually, your own self-image influences the way others see you. If you seem comfortable with your appearance, others will be too – even if there are times when you are not feeling self-assured, you can act as if you are. This can be one of the biggest challenges. Lymphoedema patients can be so conscious of how different they look that they avoid certain situations. A woman with lymphoedema of the legs was invited to a family wedding, but refused to go because she was self-conscious about her swollen limbs and the shoes she had to wear. However, with some constructive suggestions about her footwear options and about the benefits of being involved, she reconsidered. It helps to remember that it is human nature to project the aspects of ourselves that we feel good about and cover up those things we are less happy about.

SEXUALITY

Sexuality is a very important part of self-image. It is harder to enjoy physical intimacy when you do not feel confident in yourself.

Lymphoedema can cause unwelcome physical changes, which may be in addition to changes already brought about by surgery or treatment for other medical conditions. An altered body image can affect the way in which you interact with your partner, as can depression, anger and anxiety.

There are also physiological factors. Good health and fitness enhance the sexual response, whereas fatigue and illness have the opposite effect. Libido can also be affected by medication, so this should be discussed with the prescribing doctor.

When change occurs in your body and your life, you may need help in making your feelings understood. This is a time for open and honest communication, for partners to discuss realistic methods of coping. The ways of being intimate may have changed; it is important to explore new approaches to pleasing each other. It has been said that the most erotic part of the human body is the mind! The mind needs stimulation too – loving together means giving as well as receiving.

Seeking help

If you have difficulties in establishing intimacy, or in coping with any aspects of daily life, it is essential to seek help. Many people find this difficult, however, and may wait until they reach crisis point before asking for assistance. While that may be a good time for some positive action to be taken, it is important to know that you can seek help at *any* time. Having someone as a sounding board can help keep things in perspective. Successfully managing issues as they arise helps foster a sense of well-being, which is one of the keys to managing a chronic condition such as lymphoedema.

It is perfectly normal to experience a range of emotions, but these should not be allowed to interfere with the quality of everyday life. It is, on the one hand, quite understandable to feel concerned about revealing a swollen limb in public. On the other hand, if this makes you anxious about going to work or to social occasions, this is affecting your way of life and you can and should do something about it.

In the same way, while it is normal to feel low at times and to question your abilities, if you are struggling to manage ordinary tasks and have difficulty seeing a way through you may actually be suffering from depression or anxiety. Small events may become disproportionate to the extent that you retreat and become isolated.

COUNSELLING
Counselling can help you plan strategies and solutions to the challenges of daily living. It can help review your perspective, increase your sense of control and find the motivation to achieve

the physical tasks of daily living that were previously too difficult. Counselling may also help to deal with the sense of loss that so often accompanies lymphoedema and which can sometimes stop people from moving on.

Useful sources of counselling include:

- a GP
- a social worker/psychologist in a hospital or community health centre
- a breast-care nurse
- a cancer organisation
- a marriage guidance counsellor

As well as seeking the most appropriate form of support, for a therapeutic relationship to develop it is essential to feel comfortable with the counsellor.

SUPPORT GROUPS

Lymphoedema can be an isolating condition in that friends and family sometimes cannot quite comprehend the ramifications of learning to live with it. Attending a support group can provide encouragement and information. Sharing feelings and frustrations can provide much-needed support and it can be a positive experience to give something to others as well. Most support groups have guest speakers who, by sharing their knowledge and experience, have much to contribute to the outlook of group members.

However, not everyone finds support groups useful. A support group should improve the capacity to manage your condition effectively, not take from it. Some people feel disheartened or burdened down by the experiences of others, and in these situations individual help may be more appropriate.

Lymphoedema in children: one family's experience

Most people, adults and children alike, fear the unknown. Although children may be more accepting and satisfied with a simple answer, adults usually want to know how, when and why events occur. Unfortunately, there is not always a clear and simple explanation about why things happen in our lives – why, for example, some children develop lymphoedema. Despite the fact that our knowledge about lymphoedema is growing, that question still remains unanswered although geneticists are making progress in this area and the causes of secondary lymphoedema are now more clearly understood.

As parents, we eventually learnt to accept the situation when our child was diagnosed as having impaired lymph drainage. However, being informed that our son had lymphoedema was disturbing and worrying, especially as there was so little information available about the condition. The many unknowns surrounding lymphoedema are a cause of concern to many parents. Fear of the unknown can leave both parents and children feeling isolated.

There have been many stories of children who have not been correctly diagnosed for several years and of those who have received incorrect initial diagnoses. In our son's case, it took two years for lymphoedema to be diagnosed. In the beginning, we were told that he had been born deformed and would remain deformed for the rest of his life because there was nothing that could be done to help him. At the age of four, our son commenced the complex compression program (CCP) and started wearing compression garments, with great effect. The program involved massage which normally took between 15–20 minutes for each limb. Each of his fingers and toes then had to be bandaged individually and covered with padding, and a compression bandage was then applied: this process took a further fifteen to twenty minutes for each limb. Once bandaged, our son could run around the house but was unable to use his hands and therefore everything had to be done for him. The next morning we would remove the bandaging, put on his elastic stockings and gloves (easier said than done!) and then spend thirty minutes winding up his bandages ready for the next session.

We performed this routine for four months, with such good effect that his condition is now well under control. During this time, we also attended physiotherapy so that our son could do exercises. These sessions continued for many years and we still attend regular reviews. He also had laser therapy treatment several times, which, though it has not been proven as an effective treatment, was very beneficial in our case.

Although all this sounds like hard work and almost too much to cope with, as with most chronic conditions it just becomes accepted as a part of life. We are grateful that we were able to successfully control the lymphoedema and did not allow it to control us. If our son develops any swelling in the future, we will start the process all over again. He does, however, still have problems as a result of his lymph-oedema and suffers from recurring tinea and occasionally cellulitis of the knee. He also has decreased grip strength in his hands due to the slight swelling that still remains, but he learnt to touch-type at an early age and has also become quite ambidextrous.

Every child who develops lymphoedema has a different story. If lymphoedema develops at an early age, children do not know what it is like to live without it; it is part of their lives. They learn early that it is important not to pick up sharp objects such as broken glass or walk barefoot (even on the beach or in a river), because cuts can cause swelling to increase. If they do injure themselves, they know they must get treatment immediately. With younger children, however, massaging, bandaging and putting on compression gloves and stockings can be difficult.

The problems for older children with lymphoedema are more likely to be connected with self-image, particularly the desire not to be seen as different from other children. If they have to wear thick stockings or gloves, they are likely to have to continually answer questions about why they do so. In addition, a child attending a lymphoedema clinic may feel that he or she is the only child who has the condition, because most of the other people at the clinic are likely to be older. Coping with puberty and high school is also a major problem. When our son was five years old he told people that he had 'lymphoedema', which stopped them in their tracks! If people were hesitant about shaking his hand, he would say 'Oh, it won't hurt me.' But older children are more self-conscious and many have a more difficult time coping.

The support of the Lymphoedema Association during the first few years after our son's diagnosis was invaluable. Meeting other people with lymphoedema, particularly children, increased our awareness of the condition and allowed us all to learn from each other's experiences. The ability to share our concerns, successes and failures encouraged us and made us determined to share our experiences not only with those who are aware of lymphoedema, but also – importantly – with those who are not.

Nola & Geoff Brown

EIGHT

Nutrition

This chapter discusses some of the questions that are often raised about the role of nutrition in managing lymphoedema. For example, can changing the amount of protein or the type of fat in food help? The issue of weight control is also touched on, as increased and/or fluctuating weight due to swelling is a concern for many lymphoedema patients.

Any lymphoedema patient with concerns about weight gain that is not due to lymphoedema, or about nutrition, should seek the advice of an accredited practising dietitian.

The issue of weight control

Weight control is an issue for many people in the community, not just those with lymphoedema. Most of us are aware that being overweight increases our risk of developing conditions such as high blood pressure and high cholesterol, which are major risk factors in the development of heart disease and stroke. Being overweight is also associated with health problems such as diabetes.

Weight control can constitute a special challenge for people with lymphoedema, however, particularly if your condition restricts the amount of physical activity you can do. There may be psychological factors too: not only can lymphoedema cause pain and restrict movement, but a changing body shape and self-image can be distressing and depressing. Such feelings may lead to comfort eating, which can cause further weight gain. It is recommended that you discuss any such feelings with a health professional who is trained in psychology. It is important to deal with these issues rather than hope they will just go away.

THE IMPORTANCE OF DIET AND EXERCISE

In 'developed' societies the typical diet is low in fibre and high in fat, sugar, salt and alcohol. In addition, we are generally less physically active than our forebears and therefore use less energy. As a result, an increasing proportion of the population in countries such as Australia, the UK and USA is overweight.

Exercise does matter

As excessive calories and a lack of physical activity usually lead to increased body fat, it is important that lymphoedema patients take more notice of what they eat and how active they are.

Crash-dieting is not the answer

A lymphoedema patient's weight tends to fluctuate naturally as swelling comes and goes. For this reason, there is little point in weighing yourself constantly or trying to achieve some ideal weight based on a chart or a previous body size – indeed, this may well prove disheartening and counter-productive. The fact is that even losing some weight can significantly improve your health.

There is no special diet recommended for people with lymph-oedema, so it is best simply to modify eating habits in line with the dietary guidelines provided by health authorities. The Australian National Health and Medical Research Council reviews these guidelines from time to time.

'Crash' diets rarely produce long-term results. The fad diets typically reproduced in popular magazines do not take account of individual food preferences and lifestyles, and usually offer little more than rapid weight loss and lowered self-esteem if the diet fails to produce the desired outcome. While a low-calorie diet can achieve weight loss, such regimes often omit whole food groups and therefore are nutritionally unsound. Once dieting stops, weight is often regained or in some cases even increases. Similarly, skipping meals is likely to lead only to over-eating at the next meal, or over-snacking between meals. In short, it is preferable to make moderate changes to your eating habits rather than following a fad diet that may not be nutritionally adequate.

Tips for improved eating habits

It is a good idea to consult an accredited practising dietitian for further information about nutrition (food groups, serving sizes, etc.). Here are some simple suggestions for better eating habits.

- Eat a wide variety of nutritious foods.
- Start with one or two changes at a time.
- Try to include and prepare foods in a way that you will enjoy for the rest of your life, not just for a few weeks or months.
- Be comfortable with the food choices you make.
- Remember that it will take time to change old habits.
- Do not look at setbacks as failures. Perhaps the change you made was unrealistic.

Some special dietary concerns

People with lymphoedema often have questions about the part diet could play in managing their condition. These queries typically focus on three particular nutrients: protein, fat and fluids.

Protein

Some people suppose that restricting their protein intake might help lessen lymphoedema swelling. However, lymphoedema is a mechanical problem which is unaffected by the amount of protein in the lymph fluid. Proteins are the building blocks of the body's muscles and organs: the body needs protein for growth and for the repair of body tissues. There are therefore no grounds for decreasing or increasing protein intake when lymphoedema is present.

It is generally recommended that we eat 1–2 servings of meat or meat alternatives each day. One serving is equivalent to 65–100 g cooked weight of lean red meat or chicken (e.g. ½ cup of lean mince, two small or one large lamb chop, or two slices of roast meat) or 80–100 g boneless fish. Non-meat serving sizes are: two eggs (occasionally); ½ cup cooked dried (or canned) beans, lentils, chick peas or split peas; $\frac{1}{3}$ cup of peanuts or almonds, and $\frac{1}{4}$ cup sunflower or sesame seeds.

Red-meat substitutes such as poultry, fish, eggs and legumes are good sources of protein but poorer sources of iron and zinc, though these can be supplied by wholegrain or wholemeal breads and cereals. If your intake of meat or meat alternatives is below that suggested, it is recommended that you consult an accredited dietitian.

TYPES OF FAT

Polyunsaturated fats are absorbed by the intestine and pass through the lymphatic system for transport to the liver. Saturated fats, on the other hand, are absorbed by the intestine and are transported to the liver via the blood vessels. In general a diet low in fat, particularly saturated fats, is recommended because saturated fats increase the risk of heart disease.

In the 1990s, preliminary research results suggested that when treating primary lymphoedema there may be some benefit in reducing the amount of polyunsaturated fats in the diet, as this might assist lymph drainage. The study was conducted in a hospital setting, however, and there have been no conclusive results which would justify such an approach: indeed, the necessary dietary changes may be difficult to cope with in the long term.

FLUIDS

People with lymphoedema may be tempted to reduce their fluid intake as a means of reducing their swelling. This is not recommended, as water is an essential nutrient and plays a key role in the body's nutrition and the removal of waste products.

The recommended fluid intake for adults is six to eight glasses or cups of fluids per day (preferably water), unless medically directed otherwise. During hot weather, more fluid is needed to avoid dehydration or heat-stroke. Caffeinated drinks such as tea, coffee and cola have a diuretic effect (causing increased urination) and should be limited to three to four cups a day.

NINE

Foot care

The primary aim of foot care for people with lymphoedema of the legs is to maintain the body's natural defences against infection and the skin's ability to heal. Both of these attributes are compromised by lymphoedema because of the accumulation of lymph fluid in the tissue spaces, and as a result there is an increased risk that a seemingly trivial injury may develop into a more significant problem.

Many problems that affect the feet and legs can be minimised by adopting a daily foot-care regime and good general foot hygiene. It is also vital to attend to any injury promptly and to act swiftly if it becomes infected. It is important to inspect shoes daily, inside and out, for anything that might irritate or harm the feet. If your eyesight is not good, or your mobility and flexibility are limited because of arthritis or lymphoedema, a partner or carer could help.

Podiatrists are specialists in all aspects of foot care. Although there are few with a special interest in lymphoedema, all are qualified to prevent and deal with complications that may occur because of the condition. Thus, an occasional visit to a podiatrist should be part of an ongoing foot-care regime.

Basic foot-care equipment

Proper *nail clippers* are the best tools for safe and effective nail care. Scissors are usually too long and can easily nip a neighbouring toe when trimming a toenail; also, they cut by shearing through the nail, whereas clippers work more like a guillotine and so are easier to control. It is important that the jaws of the clippers meet evenly: to make sure, squeeze the handles together and check that there is no light visible through the jaws.

- A *pumice stone* is useful for keeping the skin of the feet smooth. Be careful not to rub too hard and abrade the skin.
- A *nail file* to smooth the edges of toenails after trimming is recommended to stop nails irritating adjacent toes or cutting holes in hosiery.

Before use, implements should be thoroughly cleaned of any skin or debris that might harbour germs. To do this, soak them in warm and slightly soapy water, scrub with a toothbrush, dry and then wipe with an antiseptic such as chlorhexidine solution (available from pharmacists) or methylated spirits.

Daily foot care

Daily care will do much to ensure feet are comfortable. As noted earlier, it is important that a person with lymphoedema cleans and inspects their feet daily. Wash the feet with a mild soap, taking time to clean well between the toes. It is equally important to dry the feet with a towel, especially between the toes, to help shed any loose skin that may encourage germ growth.

If you cannot reach your feet, wrap cotton gauze around the end of a ruler, dip it into methylated spirits and use this to wipe between your toes. Although less effective, you can also stand on a towel and use a hair-dryer (lowest setting) to dry the feet. As it is possible to inadvertently burn your feet with a hair-dryer, especially if your normal protective sensations have been adversely affected by lymphoedema. The sensory nerves in this area should be tested by a doctor or podiatrist to ensure that this procedure is safe.

When inspecting your feet, also check to see that toenails are not ingrowing or damaging adjacent toes. Look for corns and calluses (see page 92) on the balls of the feet and the sides of the toes, and for any cracks in the skin, particularly around the heels. Check also for any possible sites of infection, including mosquito bites and gardening cuts and scratches. (See also 'Dealing with common foot infections on page 93.)

TOENAILS

Generally speaking, nails should be trimmed straight across and not too short, leaving about a millimetre of free nail (Figures 9.1 and 9.2). The corners should be gently rounded so that they do not catch on hosiery or an adjacent toe. Toenails that are difficult to cut because they are too wide (Figure 9.3), too curved (Figure 9.4) and/or too thick (Figure 9.5) usually require professional attention. Although abnormal toenails may be present at birth, distorted growth of the nail usually results from long-forgotten damage to the toes, even shoes that are too short or tight.

It is possible for corns to form at the edges of a toenail as a result of constant pressure being exerted by the margins of the nail against the toe. This can cause the toenail to become very sore. Often, trimming the nail will reveal a blister or corn beneath

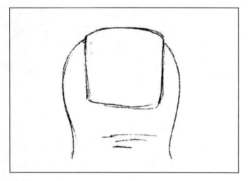

Figure 9.1 Top view of a normal toenail.

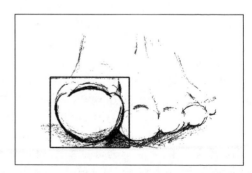

Figure 9.2 Front view of a normal toenail with only a gentle curve from side to side.

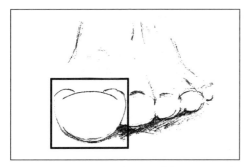

Figure 9.3 Front view of a toenail that is too wide for the toe. Notice how the edges of the toe (sulci) overlap the nail.

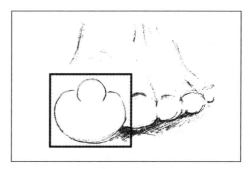

Figure 9.4 Front view of a toenail that is too curved (incurvated) for the toe. Notice how the edges of the toe (sulci) overlap the nail.

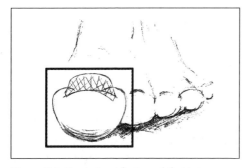

Figure 9.5 Front view of a toenail that is too thick (onychauxic) or too deformed (onchogryphosis).

it which may require the care of a podiatrist.

Occasionally a fungal infection will cause a toenail to become distorted. This can also be the cause of a great deal of discomfort underneath the nail itself because of the build-up of a callus associated with the fungi.

Sometimes the toenails (and fingernails) of people with lymphoedema can become slow-growing, thickened and yellow – known as the yellow nail syndrome. This is because the long-term presence of swelling can affect the health of the nail bed (where the nail grows from) and change the nails' growth pattern.

Ingrowing nails

If lymphoedema of the lower limb causes the toes to swell, the skin of the toe will press against the nail. In these cases, the nails should be cut short at the sides: this is best done by a podiatrist, because extra care must be taken to ensure that the nail has no rough edges which might dig into the skin and cause an ingrowing toenail, which can easily become infected (Figures 9.6 and 9.7).

It can be tempting to treat ingrowing toenails with special products designed to soften the nail. These preparations should be avoided because they can damage the surrounding skin and so increase the risk of a more serious injury. Sometimes it is necessary for a recurrently ingrowing toenail to be reshaped permanently through minor surgery, which is usually performed under local anaesthesia: a podiatrist or doctor can advise about this.

Talcum and foot powders

Powders are not a substitute for correct drying and should be used sparingly, if at all, on the feet. Most people use powders very liberally: if powder is not removed from between the toes, it can quickly accumulate and, together with moisture, form the ideal environment for germs to grow.

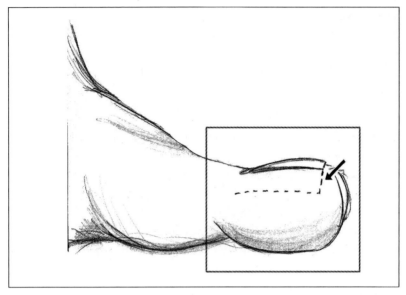

Figure 9.6 Side view. Note the overlap of the edges of the toenail by the edges of the toe (sulci).

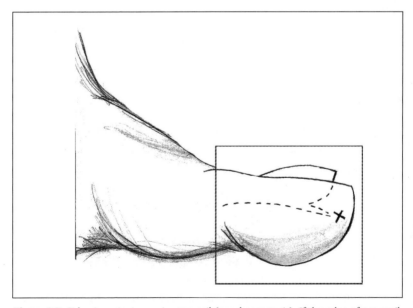

Figure 9.7 Side view. An ingrowing toe nail (onychocryptosis). If the edge of a toenail is cut too short or if the edge of the toe (sulci) overlaps the nail, any ragged edge may grow into the skin and an infection occur.

FOOT EXERCISES

Swelling of the legs can lead to reduced movement at the ankle joint, which is often signalled by an increased tendency to catch the toes when walking and stumble on the slightest underfoot irregularity. Exercises to correct this stiffness are vital and the best are those used as a warm-up by joggers.

1. Stand on one foot with the knee straight and lean forward, bending only at the ankle, supporting yourself against a wall. Hold this position for 15 seconds, until you notice a tight feeling in the calf just below the knee. Rest the toes of the other foot on the ground for balance.
2. Then, keeping the foot flat to the ground, bend that knee forward until the tightness shifts to the Achilles tendon just behind the ankle. Hold this position for 15 seconds.

Even if the swelling and stiffness are only in one leg, this cycle should be repeated three times for both legs, morning and night. It is important to be patient, as it will be at least a month before there is a noticeable improvement. A podiatrist or physiotherapist can advise about this and suggest other exercises to help improve mobility.

Corns and calluses

Calluses are caused by the top skin layer thickening to protect itself from intermittent but repetitive pressure (e.g. from a shoe). Corns are calluses that have thickened even more because of the continued irritation of the skin over a bony prominence of the foot. Occasionally, blisters or small ulcers can form underneath corns. Provided problems such as these are recognised quickly, some simple first-aid procedures (see page 97) will greatly reduce the risk of further complications.

Corns and calluses on the sole of the foot usually develop as a consequence of how we walk, and will form on the parts of the feet that are more stable and so carry more of the body weight when walking. Corns can form on the tops and sides of toes if shoe uppers are too tight, especially on prominent bunions or claw toes. Less serious cases can be managed successfully by a podiatrist, through regular foot care.

For the most serious cases, surgery can be used to smooth any underlying bony prominence and so minimise the internal high points of pressure. Padding can be used to reduce pressure on the feet caused by shoes during walking. But it is important to remember that with lymphoedema of the feet there is little room to spare inside a shoe for even the thinnest insoles available in pharmacies and supermarkets; a walking shoe with a soft midsole may offer greater cushioning.

If a callus in the heel area thickens too quickly, splits can occur which may be very painful and provide an entry point for infections. A heel callus should be removed by a podiatrist and steps must be taken to ensure that the splits do not progress too deeply. It is advisable to avoid wearing shoes which allow the heel of the foot to overhang the shoe heel, as the skin can thicken and crack very quickly.

DAY-TO-DAY CARE

Use a pumice stone daily on corns and calluses, preferably after a bath or shower, with a little soap when the foot is still wet. The aim is to keep the skin soft, smooth, resilient and healthy, so a cream (e.g. sorbitol) should also be applied daily. Drying well between the toes with a towel and methylated spirits should also become a habit. Razor blades and chemical corn cures should not be used, because this creates a greater risk of infection at the site.

Off-the-shelf corn preparations are not recommended. Not only can the chemicals in these products cause considerable skin damage with little warning pain, but healthy skin may be accidentally burned because it is difficult to stop the solution spreading.

Dealing with common foot infections

Infections of the feet may be fungal, viral or bacterial in origin. Tinea (athlete's foot) is a fungal infection, and warts (*verrucae pedis*, or papillomas) result from a virus. Bacterial infections can be serious because they can cause the spreading skin infection called cellulitis. While the most common entry point for a bacterial skin infection is between the toes when tinea is present, any break in the skin can allow an infection to enter. The importance of recognising and treating even minor injuries cannot be over-emphasised.

VIRAL INFECTIONS

Viral infections such as warts are difficult to treat because doing so involves destroying the skin cells that contain the virus. Usually the treatment (chemicals, cryotherapy or freezing, or surgical removal) causes more discomfort than the wart itself. Therefore prevention – taking time to carefully wash and dry the feet regularly – is the best cure. Wipe the feet daily with methylated spirits, especially after using public facilities such as pools and showers, to minimise the risk of catching secondary infections. There is little point wearing shoes or thongs in public pools because water containing infected skin cells can still wash over your feet, and anyway there is a much greater risk of slipping and falling over in such footwear.

TINEA

If the presence of tinea is suspected and you are confident you are drying your feet properly, an anti-fungal preparation should be applied daily: antifungal agents, available from pharmacists, include clotrimozole, miconazole and econozole. If the tinea is very resistant or the toenails develop a fungal infection, anti-fungal tablets such as terbinafine may be prescribed.

Choosing footwear

People with or without lymphoedema require the same features in a shoe. The ideal shoe has a stable heel counter (the firm section that wraps around the heel of the foot), which encourages the foot to remain correctly positioned. A shoe should also bend freely at the point where the toes bend at the ball of the foot (Figure 9.8). Finally, of course, the shoe should feel right when worn. If you compare the feet of a group of people, some appear straight while some curve one way and others curve another: naturally, the most comfortable shoe will be one where the shape of the last closely matches the shape of the foot.

STYLE AND FIT

It was long believed that bunions and claw toes were caused by poorly fitting shoes. It is now recognised that although shoes can aggravate these conditions they are rarely the prime cause. It is, however, important to wear shoes that fit well and are the right style for the circumstances, such as proper walking shoes for long walks. If, on the other hand, you are going out and want to wear high-fashion shoes that are not very comfortable, try to wear them for as short a time as possible (e.g. wear more comfortable shoes to and from the event and change into the 'party' shoes on arrival).

It is also important to bear in mind that a shoe might be the perfect size but the style may be wrong for your foot; larger shoes in the same style will not solve the problem, as it may be necessary to curl the toes to hold the shoes on, which will only exacerbate the original problem.

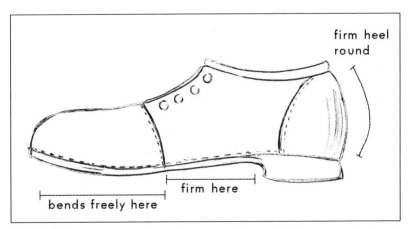

Figure 9.8 Some of the important features of a shoe that will help improve the function of your feet. The shoes should also fit your feet well.

If necessary, a bootmaker or shoe repairer can stretch shoes to accommodate misshapen toes, bunions, etc. This can also be done at home, using a broom: place the broom upright (handle pointing skyward) and meanwhile locate the tight spot in the shoe by rubbing a finger slowly along the inside of the upper. Then place the shoe over the end of the broom and gently rock it from side to side at the pressure point for about 30 minutes, which will gently stretch the leather in that spot. (Trying to stretch the upper too quickly may cause the leather to split.) This procedure will only work if there is no stitching across the pressure point, because stitching will not stretch.

CORRECT SUPPORT FOR THE FEET

Shoes not only protect the sole of the foot from the surface you walk on, but are also intended to enhance 'normal' foot motion. The foot generally functions best when it is positioned immediately beneath the leg, so always look for shoes which keep your foot from rolling too far inwards or outwards. Many of the aches and pains that afflict the feet and legs can be attributed to the motion of the foot being less than ideal, which puts extra strain on the foot ligaments and the muscles that supply the feet as they struggle to stabilise their many bones when standing and walking. Naturally, these aches are greater if the legs are heavier due to lymphoedema swelling. Obviously, reducing the lymphoedema should be a priority, as apart from anything else this will make the legs lighter to carry.

Shoes that cover the instep and can be adjusted (e.g. by laces or Velcro fastenings) to accommodate the swelling are best. If feet swell, wearing low-cut shoes for walking is not a good idea: even if a compression garment is worn, the top of your foot may bulge over the sides of the shoe, which can irritate and damage the foot.

There are times when it is necessary to supplement well-fitting and supportive shoes with specialised supports (called orthoses) to keep the feet in the best possible position. These inserts are designed to compensate for alignment problems of the lower limb, such as bow legs, knock knees or flat feet, which can otherwise make walking uncomfortable.

Compression garments

It is best to avoid wearing tight compression garments over the toes. The garment can be cut at this end so that the toes do not rub together – their doing so can have the same effect as leaving a dressing on for too long and can even cause corns on the sides of the small toes. Any alterations to a compression garment are best supervised by a therapist or podiatrist.

First aid

Any injury to the foot should be cleaned with water and then flushed with warm salty water ($\frac{1}{2}$ cup salt to a 9-litre bucket of water).

Initially, only a mild antiseptic (such as chlorhexidine cream) should be used, because stronger antiseptics can delay healing by hampering the body's cell repair processes.

Lightweight, hypo-allergenic dressings such as Cutiplast or Hansapor are ideal because the adhesive is not too strong and the risks of an allergic reaction are small. Whatever type of dressing is used, it is important not to leave it on for too long as this can cause the skin to become white, soft and prune-like, and therefore more susceptible to secondary infections.

References

Chapter 2: Lymphoedema

Evans, A.L., Brice, G., Sotirova, V., Mortimer, P., Beninson, J., Burnand, K., Rosbotham, J., Child, A., Safarazi, M. Mapping of primary lymphoedema to the 5q35.3 region. *American Journal of Human Genetics* **64**, 547–55, 1999.

Fang, J., Dagenais, S.L., Erickson, R.P., Arlt, M.F., Glynn, M.W., Gorski, J.L., Seaver, L.H. and Glover T.W. Mutations in FOXC2 (MFH-1), a forkhead family transcription factor, are responsible for the hereditary lymphedema-distichiasis syndrome. *American Journal of Human Genetics* **67**, 1382–8, 2000.

Ferrell, R.E., Levinson, K.L., Esman, J.H., Kimak, M.A., Lawrence, E.C., Barmada, M.M., Finegold, D.N. Hereditary lymphedema: evidence for linkage and genetic heterogeneity. *Human Molecular Genetics* **7**, 2073–8, 1998.

Karkkainen, M.J., Ferrell, R.E., Lawrence, E.C., Kimak, M.A., Levinson, K.L., McTigue, M.A., Alitalo, K., Finegold, D.N. Missense mutations interfere with VEGFR-3 signalling in primary lymphoedema. *Nature Genetics* **25**, 153–9, 2000.

Mangion, J., Rahman, N., Mansour, S., Brice, G., Rosbotham, J., Child, A.H., Murday, V.A., Mortimer, P.S., Barfoot, R., Sigurdsson, A., Edkins, S., Sarfarazi, M., Burnand, K., Evans, A.L., Nunan, T.O., Stratton, M.R., Jeffery, S. A gene for lymphedema-distichiasis maps to 16q24.3. *American Journal of Human Genetics* **65**, 427–32, 1999.

Witte, M.H., Erickson, R., Bernas, M., Andrade, M., Reiser F., Conlon, W., Hoyme, H.E., Witte, C.L. Phenotypic and genotypic heterogeneity in familial lymphedema. *Lymphology* **31**, 145–55, 1998.

Chapter 3: Approaches to managing lymphoedema

Bernas, M.J., Witte, C.L. and M.H. The diagnosis and treatment of peripheral lymphedema: Draft revision of the 1995 consensus document of the international society of lymphology executive committee for discussion at the September 3–7,2001, XVIII. *Lymphology* **34**, 84–91, 2001.

Burt, J., White, G. *Lymphedema: A breast cancer patient's guide to prevention and healing.* California: Hunter House, 1999.

Földi, M. Treatment of Lymphedema. *Lymphology* **27**, 1–5, 1994.

Földi, M. Massage and damage to lymphatics. *Lymphology* **28**, 1–3, 1995.

Kurz, I. *Introduction to Dr Vodder's Manual Lymph Drainage.* Volume 3: *Therapy II (Treatment Manual),* 57–69. Heidelberg: Karl F. Hauf, 1987.

Swirsky, J., Sackett-Nannery, D. *Coping with lymphedema: A practical guide to understanding, treating, and living with lymphedema.* New York: Avery Publishing Group, 1998.

Witte, C.L. and M.H. Consensus and Dogma. **31**, 98–100, 1998.

Wittlinger, H. and G. *Textbook of Dr Vodder's Manual Lymph Drainage.* Volume 1: Basic Course, 25–35. Heidelberg: Karl F. Hauf, 1987.

Chapter 4: The role of exercise in lymphoedema management

NHMRC *Physical Activity Guidelines for Australians.* Canberra: Australian Government Publishing Service, 1998.

NHMRC *Dietary Guidelines for Older Australians.* Canberra: Australian Government Publishing Service, 1999.

Brennan, M.J. and Miller, L.T. Overview of treatment options and review of the current role and use of compression garments, intermittent pumps, and exercise in the management of lymph-oedema. *Cancer* Supplement **83** (No. 12), 1998.

Carter, B.J. Women's experiences of lymphoedema. Oncology Nursing Forum **24** (No. 5), 875–81, 1997.

Casley-Smith, J.R. Modern treatment of lymphoedema. Modern Medicine of Australia **35** No. 5, 70–83, May 1992.

Clark, R., Wasilewska, T. & Carter, J. Lymphoedema: a study of Otago women treated for breast cancer. *Nursing Praxis in New Zealand*, **12** (No. 2), 4–15, 1997.

Dimeo, F.C., Stieglitz, R.D., Novelli-Fischer, U., Fetscher, S., Keul, J. Effects of physical activity on the fatigue and psychologic status of cancer patients during chemotherapy. *Cancer* **89** (No. 10), 2273–7, 1999.

Dimeo, F.C., Rumberger B., Keul, J. Aerobic exercise as therapy for cancer fatigue. *Medicine and Science in Sports and Exercise* Vol. 30, No. 4, 475–8, 1998.

Fiatarone, M., Marks, E.C., Ryan, N.D., Meredith, C.N., Lipsitz, L.A., Evans, W.J. High-intensity strength training in nonagenarians. *Journal of the American Medical Association* Vol. **263**, No. 22, 3029–3034, June 1990.

Földi, E. and M., Clodius, L. The lymphoedema chaos: A Lancet. *Annals of Plastic Surgery*, **22** (No. 6), 505–515, 1989.

Földi, M. and E. *Lymphoedema: Methods of Treatment and Control – a Guide for Patients and Therapists* (English translation). 1993. Victoria, Australia.

Hwang, J.H., Kwon, J.Y., Lee, K.W., Choi, J.Y., Kim, B.T., Lee, B.B., Kim, D.I. Changes in lymphatic function after complex physical therapy for lymphoedema. *Lymphology* **32**, 15–21, 1999.

Kent, H. Breast cancer survivors begin to challenge exercise taboos. *Canadian Medical Association Journal*, **155** (No. 7), 1996, 969–971.

Lord, S., Castell, S. Effect of exercise on balance, strength and reaction time in older people. *Australian Physiotherapy* Vol **40**, No. 2, 83–87, 1994.

Mortimer, P.S. Managing lymphoedema. *Clinical and Experimental Dermatology* **20**, 98–106, 1995.

Nelson, M.E. *Strong Women Stay Young*. Thomas C. Lothian Pty Ltd, Melbourne, 1997.

Nelson, M.E. *Strong Women Stay Slim*. Thomas C. Lothian Pty Ltd, Melbourne, 1998.

Chapter 5: Compression therapy, laser therapy and compression pumps

Bringezu, G., Schreiner, O. *Die Therapieform Manuelle Lymphdrainage*, 342–4. Lübeck: Ebert Verlag, 1991. Not available in English.

Casley-Smith, J. and J.R. *Modern Treatment for Lymphoedema*, 201–2. Adelaide: The Lymphoedema Association of Australia, 1994.

Földi, M.E. *Das Lymphödem Vorbeugung und Behandlung*, 94–6. München: Urban & Fischer, 1999. Not available in English.

Földi, M., Kubik, S. *Lehrbuch der Lymphologie für Mediziner und Physiotherapeuten*. p. 315. Stuttgart: Gustav Fischer, 1999. Not available in English.

Kurz, I. *Introduction to Dr Vodder's Manual Lymph Drainage*. Volume 3: *Therapy II (Treatment Manual)*, 21–48. Heidelberg: Karl F. Hauf, 1987.

Mason, M. *Living with Lymphoedema: A Handbook for Patients*, 27–8. Adelaide: Norwood Lymphoedema Clinic, 1995.

Piller, N. Lymphoedema rehabilitation programme. *The European Journal of Lymphology and Related Problems* **13** (No. 11), 60–2, 1992.

Piller, N. The management and treatment of lymphoedema. *National Women's Health Group Journal* **13**, 21, 1994.

Weissleder, H., Schuchhardt, C. (eds). *Lymphedema Diagnosis and Treatment*, 270–2. Bonn: Kagerer Kommunikation, 1997.

Chapter 6: Surgery and drug therapy

Alder, S. Guidelines for the surgical management of breast cancer: comment. *Australian and New Zealand Journal of Surgery* **69**, 748, 1999.

Baumeister, R., Siuda, S., Bohmert, H. and Moser, E. A microsurgical method for reconstruction of interrupted lymphatic pathway: autologous lymph-vessel transplantation for treatment of lymphedemas. *Scandinavian Journal of Plastic and Reconstructive Surgery and Hand Surgery* **20**, 141–6, 1986.

Brorson, H., Svensson, H. Complete reduction of lymphoedema

of the arm by liposuction after breast cancer. *Scandinavian Journal of Plastic and Reconstructive Surgery and Hand Surgery* **31**, 137–43, 1997.

Brorson, H. and Svensson, H. Liposuction combined with controlled compression therapy reduces arm lymphedema more effectively than controlled compression therapy alone. *Plastic and Reconstructive Surgery* **102**, 1058–67, 1998.

Brorson, H. Liposuction gives complete reduction of chronic large arm lymphedema after breast cancer. *Acta Oncologica* **39**, 407–20, 2000.

Brorson, H., Svensson, H. Skin blood flow of the lymphademat- ous arm before and after liposuction. *Lymphology* **31**, 165–72, 1997.

Campisi, C., Boccardo, F., Zilli, A., Maccio, A., Napoli, F. Long- term results after lymphatic-venous anastomoses for the treatment of obstructive lymphedema. *Microsurgery* **21**, 135–9, 2001.

Campisi, C., Boccardo, F., Zilli, A., Maccio, A., Napoli, F. The use of vein grafts in the treatment of peripheral lymphedemas: long-term results. *Microsurgery* **21**, 143–7, 2001.

Gilbert, A., O'Brien, B., Vorrath, J., Sykes, P. Lymphaticovenous anastomosis by microvascular technique. *British Journal of Plastic Surgery* **29**, 355–60, 1976.

Huang, G., Hu, R., Liu, Z. Microlymphaticovenous anastomosis in the treatment of lower limb obstructive lymphedema: analysis of 91 cases. *Plastic and Reconstructive Surgery* **76**, 671–7, 1985.

Knight, K., Khazanchi, R., Pederson, W. *et al.* Coumarin and 7-hydroxycoumarin treatment of canine obstructive lymph- oedema. *Clinical Science* **77**, 69–76, 1989.

Koshima, I., Inagawa, K., Urushibara, K., Moriguchi, T. Super- microsurgical lymphaticovenular anastomosis for the treatment of lymphedema in the upper extremities. *Journal of Recon- structive Microsurgery* **16**, 437–42, 2000.

Miller, T., Wyatt, L. and Rudkin, G. Staged skin and subcutaneous excision for lymphedema: a favorable report of long-term results. *Plastic and Reconstructive Surgery* **102**, 1486–98, 1998.

Morrison, W. Lymphoedema: the role of microlymphatic surgery vs. debulking procedures. *Perspectives in Vascular Surgery* **3**, 142–62, 1990.

O'Brien, B., Mellow, C., Zhazanchi, R. *et al.* Long-term results after lymphatovenous anastomoses for the treatment of obstructive lymphedema. *Plastic and Reconstructive Surgery* **85**, 562–72, 1990.

O'Brien, B. and Morrison, W. *Reconstructive Microsurgery.* Edinburgh: Churchill Livingstone, 1987.

Pain, S., Purushotham, A. Lymphoedema following surgery for breast cancer. *British Journal of Surgery* **87**, 1128–41, 2000.

Piller, N., Morgan, R., Casley-Smith, J.R. A double-blind, cross-over trial of 0-(beta-hydroxyethyl)-rutosides (benzopyrones) in the treatment of lymphoedema of the arms and legs. *British Journal of Plastic Surgery* **41**, 20–7, 1988.

Puckett, C., Jacobs, G., Hurvitz, J., Silver, D. Evaluation of lymphovenous anastomosis in obstructive lymphoedema. *Plastic and Reconstructive Surgery* **66**, 116–20, 1980.

Yamamoto, Y., Sugihara, T. Microsurgical lymphaticovenous implantation for the treatment of chronic lymphedema. *Plastic and Reconstructive Surgery* **101**, 157–61, 1998.

Chapter 7: Psychological and lifestyle considerations

Carter, B. Women's experiences of lymphoedema. *Cancer Nursing* **24** (No. 5), 875–881, 1997.

Passik, S. and McDonald, M. Psychosocial Aspects of Upper Extremity Lymphedema in Women Treated for Breast Cancer. New York: American Cancer Society Lymphoedema Workshop, 1998. Reprints available from Steven Passik, 115 West 19th St Indianapolis IN 46202.

Passik, S., Newman, M., Brennan, M. and Holland, J. Psychiatric consultation for women undergoing rehabilitation for upper-extremity lymphoedema following breast cancer treatment. *Journal of Pain and Symptom Management* **8**, 226–33, 1993.

Passik, S., Newman, M., Brennan, M. and Tunkel, R. Predictors of psychological distress, sexual dysfunction and physical functioning among women with upper extremity lymphedema related to breast cancer. *Psycho-Oncology* **4**, 255–63, 1995.

Rose, K. An issue of powerlessness: psychosocial issues affecting breast cancer care. *Professional Nurse*, 434–8, April, 1994. Breast

Woods, M. Sociological factors and psychosocial implications of lymphoedema. *International Journal of Palliative Nursing* **1** (No. 1), 17–20, 1995.

Chapter 8: Nutrition

Smith, A., Kellet, E., Schmerlaib, Y. *The Australian Guide to Healthy Eating.* Commonwealth Department of Health and Family Services: Children's Health Development Foundation (South Australia). Commonwealth of Australia, 1998.

Soria, P., Cuesta, A., Romero, H., Martinez, F.J., Sastre, A. Dietary treatment of lymphoedema by restriction of long-chain triglycerides. *Angiology* **45**(8), 703–7, 1994.

Resources

This section lists useful contacts and organisations around the world. As addresses and telephone numbers may change, we recommend that you check the latest directory. Numbers with the prefix 13 can be called from anywhere in Australia for the price of a local call.

Lymphoedema support

AUSTRALIA

A number of these organisations will have a list of lymphoedema practitioners

ACT Lymphoedema Support Group
19 Bardsley Place
Holt ACT 2615 Australia
Tel: 61 2 6254 4753
Email: geoff.moore@bigpond.com

Darwin Lymphoedema Support Group
Cancer Council of NT
PO Box 42719
Casuarina NT 0811
Tel: 61 8 89 27 4888
Email: supportw@ozemail.com.au

Lymphoedema Support Group of South Australia Inc
PO Box 1006
Kent Town SA 5071 Australia
Tel: 61 8 83367748
Email: bartel.Maureen@sagov.sa.gov.au

Lymphoedema Association of Victoria Inc
PO Box 2412
Nth Ringwood Vic. 3134 Australia
Tel: 1300 852 850
Email: info@lav.org.au
Website: www.lav.org.au

Lymphoedema Support Group of NSW
204/ 5-9 Everton St
Pymble NSW 2073 Australia
Tel: 61 2 9402 5625
Email: basmith1@bigpond.com

Lymphoedema Association of Queensland Inc
PO Box 3068
Bracken Ridge QLD 4017 Australia
Tel: 61 7 3269 1498
Fax: 61 7 3269 1498
Email: lymphqld@powerup.com.au
Website: www.powerup.com.au/~lymphqld

Tasmania Lymphoedema Support Group
c/o 42 Stanley Street
Bellerive Hobart Tas. 7018 Australia
Tel & Fax: 61 3 6244 4634

Lymphoedema Association of Western Australia
PO Box 2037
Claremont North WA 6010 Australia
Tel: 61 8 9276 8397

Other lymphoedema organisations

AUSTRALIA

Australasian Lymphology Association (for health professionals)
PO Box 1879
Milton QLD 4064 Australia
Tel: 1300 132 962
Email: bmirolo@hoca.com.au

Lymphoedema Association of Australia Inc
Dr Judy Casley-Smith (Chairperson)
94 Cambridge Terrace, Malvern
SA 5061 Australia
Tel: 61 8 8271 2198
Fax: 61 8 8271 8776
Email: casley@internode.on.net.com.au
Website: http://www.lymphoedema.org.au

USA

The National Lymphedema Network
1611 Telegraph Avenue, Suite 1111
Oakland CA 94612
Tel: 0011 1 510 208 3200
Email: nln@lymphnet.org
Website: www.lymphnet.org

International Society of Lymphology (for health professionals)
Central office:
M.H. Witte, MD, Sec. Gen'l, International Society of Lymphology
& Professor of Surgery
University of Arizona College of Medicine
Department of Surgery (GS&T)
P.O. Box 245063, 1501 N
Campbell Avenue
Tucson, Arizona 85724-5063 USA
Tel: 0011 1 520 626-6118
Email: lymph@u.arizona.edu
Website: www.u.arizona.edu/~witte/ISL.htm

The North American Vodder Association of Lymphatic Therapy (NAVALT)
1140 Turbin Road
Inman, SC 29349 USA
Tel: 0011 1 888 462- 8258
Fax: 0011 1 972 243-3227
Website: www.navalt.com

UK

British Lymphology Society
1 Webb's Court, Buckhurst Avenue
Sevenoaks Kent TN13 1LZ UK
Tel: 0011 44 1732 740850
Fax: 0011 44 1732 459225
Email: helensnoad@blsac.demon.co.uk
Website: www.lymphoedema.org/bls

Lymphoedema Support Network (LSN)
St. Luke's Crypt
Sydney Street
London
SW3 6NH
Tel: 0011 44 20 7351 4480
Fax: 0011 44 20 7349 0909
Email: adminlsn@lymphoedema.freeserve.co.uk
Website: http://www.lymphoedema.org/lsn

Cancer

Helpline 13 11 20 (All Cancer Councils in Australia)

CANCER COUNCILS IN AUSTRALIA

The Cancer Council ACT
159 Maribyrnong Avenue
Kaleen ACT 2617 Australia
Tel: 61 2 6262 2222
Fax: 61 2 6262 2223
Email: reception@actcancer.org
Website: www.actcancer.org

The Cancer Council New South Wales
153 Dowling Street
Woolloomooloo NSW 2011 Australia
Tel: 61 2 9334 1900
Fax: 61 2 9358 1452
Email: feedback@cancercouncil.com.au
Website: www.cancercouncil.com.au

The Cancer Council Northern Territory
P.O. Box 42719
Casuarina NT 0811 Australia
Tel: 61 8 8927 4888
Fax: 61 8 8927 4990
Email: uvstop@cancernt.org.au
Website: www.cancercouncilnot.com.au

The Cancer Council Tasmania
140 Bathurst Street
Hobart Tas. 7000 Australia
Tel: 61 3 6233 2030
Fax: 61 3 6233 2123
Email: infotas@cancer.org.au
Website: www.cancer.org.au/tas/

The Cancer Council Victoria
1 Rathdowne Street
Carlton Sth Vic. 3053 Australia
Tel: 61 3 9635 5000
Fax: 61 3 9635 5270
Email: enquiries@cancervic.org.au
Website: www.cancervic.org.au

Cancer Council South Australia
202 Greenhill Road
Eastwood SA 5063 Australia
Tel: 61 8 8291 4111
Fax: 61 8 8291 4122
Email: tcc@cancersa.org.au
Website: www.cancersa.org.au

Cancer Foundation of Western Australia
46 Ventnor Avenue
West Perth WA 6005 Australia
Tel: 61 8 9212 4333
Fax: 61 8 9212 4399
Email: cancerwa@cancerwa.asn.au
Website: www.education@cancerwa.asn.au

Queensland Cancer Fund
553 Gregory Terrace
Fortitude Valley Qld 4006
Tel: 61 7 3258 2200
Fax: 61 7 3257 1306
Email: qldcf@qldcancer.com.au
Website: www.qldcancer.com.au

OTHER AUSTRALIAN CANCER ORGANISATIONS
Breast Cancer Network Australia
PO Box 4082
Auburn South Vic. 3122 Australia
Tel: 61 3 9805 2500
Fax: 61 3 9805 2599
Email: beacon@bcna.org.au
Website: www.bcna.org.au

National Breast Cancer Centre
Locked Bag 16
Kings Cross NSW 1340 Australia
Tel: 61 2 9036 3030
Fax: 61 2 9036 3077
Email: directorate@nbcc.org.au
Website: www.nbc.org.au

National Breast Cancer Foundation
Suite 402, 90 Pitt Street
Sydney NSW 2000 Australia
Tel: 61 2 9235 3444
Fax: 61 2 9233 3442
Email: nbcfl@nbcf.org.au
Web site: www.nbcf.org.au

NEW ZEALAND

The Auckland Lymphoedema Support Network will provide contact details for other divisions upon enquiry.

Lymphoedema Support Network—Auckland
c/– Auckland Cancer Society
P.O. Box 1724
Auckland
New Zealand
Tel: 0011 64 9 308 0162 or Joy Donohoe 0011 64 9 625 6463
Email: donohofam@ihug.co.nz
Cancer Information Service—0800 800 426

Nutrition

Nutrition Society of Australia
PO Box 949
Kent Town SA 5071 Australia
Tel: 61 8 8363 1307
Fax: 61 8 8363 1604
Email: info@nsa.asn.au
Website: www.nsa.asn.au/links.html
'The Australian Guide to Healthy Eating' poster, a booklet and background information is available from the Publications Officer, Public Health Division, Department of Health and Ageing and Family Services
Tel (toll-free): 1 800 020 103, ext. 8654
Email: phd.publications@health.gov.au
Website: www.health.gov.au/pubhlth/strateg/food/guide/

Podiatry

Australasian Podiatry Council
41 Derby Street
Collingwood Vic. 3066 Australia
Tel: 61 3 9416 3111
Fax: 61 3 9416 3188
Email: apodc@ozemail.com.au
Website: www.apodc.com.au

Glossary

AIDS Acquired immune deficiency syndrome, caused by the human immunodeficiency virus (HIV).

antibiotics Drugs or other substances that destroy or inhibit the growth of microorganisms (bacteria).

antibodies Various proteins produced in the body to counteract toxins and other unwanted foreign substances.

axilla (also called the armpit) The space under the shoulder between the upper part of the arm and the side of the chest.

axillary clearance A surgical procedure involving removal of lymph nodes in the armpit.

bio-impedance meter An instrument which passes a small amount of electrical current through selected regions of the body and can measure the amount of fluid accumulating between the cells. A useful tool for measuring oedema.

blood pressure The pressure exerted by the blood on the walls of blood vessels. Abnormally high blood pressure is known as hypertension; low blood pressure is called hypotension.

capillaries The smallest blood vessels, which link the arteries and the veins. The site where oxygen and nutrients leave the blood to nourish the tissues and where most waste products are taken up.

cellulitis An inflammation of the skin or subcutaneous tissue resulting from a bacterial infection. People with lymphoedema are prone to recurrent episodes of cellulitis. *See also* erysipelas and lymphangitis.

compression garment A tightly knit elastic stocking or sleeve designed to apply pressure to part of the body to slow the flow of fluid from the vascular system into the tissue of a limb.

congenital Medical condition present at birth.

dermal back-flow The movement of fluids from the larger lymph vessels into the smaller ones, from which the fluid then leaks out into the tissue spaces.

diabetes mellitus A disorder of carbohydrate metabolism as a result of disturbances in insulin production from the pancreas.

distal Farthest from the point of attachment or origin: for example, the knee is distal to the hip.

diuretic Drugs or other substances promoting the production of urine.

endocrine system (also called the hormone system) The system of ductless glands, including the thyroid, which secrete hormones into the bloodstream and stimulate the various parts of the body to carry out their functions.

erysipelas Infection of the skin and subcutaneous tissues due to a *streptococcal infection*.

fibrosis The spreading of fibre-like (fibrous) tissue.

genes The biologic unit of heredity.

hyperplasia An abnormal increase in the number of lymph vessels in an organ or tissue.

hypo-parathyroidism An auto-immune condition produced by greatly reduced function of the parathyroid glands, or following their removal.

immune system The intricate system by which the body defends itself against infection. It includes the lymph nodes and other structures.

latent or hidden phase In lymphoedema, a stage during which there are changes to the fibre and fluids in tissue but the size of the limb is not affected.

lipoedema A condition seen predominantly in women, characterised by abnormal deposits of adipose (fatty) tissue, especially in the legs.

liposuction A surgical technique for the removal of unwanted subcutaneous fat.

lumpectomy The surgical removal of a breast tumour and a small area of surrounding tissue.

lymphatic system A complex network of vessels which collects, filters and carries away excess fluid from the tissues and plays an important part in the body's immune system.

lymph The clear, colourless fluid (composed mainly of water and proteins, waste products and white blood cells) carried in the lymphatic vessels. Originating in the spaces between the cells in tissues (where it is called extracellular fluid), lymph is pumped through the lymphatic system towards lymph nodes.

lymph nodes Small structures (about 1500 in all) located throughout the body, which filter lymph and produce antibodies and lymphocytes if foreign substances are detected.

lymphangitis An inflammation of the walls of the major lymph vessels, in response to the presence of bacteria or toxins.

lymphatic trunk (more correctly called lymph collectors) The larger lymphatic vessels.

lymphocyte A type of white blood cell formed in lymphatic tissue. A vital constituent of the immune system, lymphocytes fight infection and promote wound healing.

lymphoedema A swelling initially caused by an accumulation of fluid in the tissues when the lymphatic system fails to remove it. Later the protein-rich fluid is replaced by fibres which cause the affected tissue to harden. **Primary lymphoedema** is associated with a genetic abnormality. **Secondary lymphoedema** occurs when the lymphatic system is damaged or destroyed by surgery, radiation therapy or some other trauma.

lymphoscintigram A diagnostic technique that creates a 3-D picture of lymph vessels and shows the functional status of a lymphatic system.

lymphovenous anastomosis A connection (formed spontaneously or surgically) between a large lymph collector and a small vein, through which fluids can move easily.

macrophage A large white blood cell that clears away microorganisms and other unwanted foreign particles in the body.

magnetic resonance imaging (MRI) A diagnostic technique used to assess structural changes in tissue, such as enlarged lymph nodes and abnormalities of the circulatory system.

manual lymphatic drainage A massage technique used to move lymphatic fluid from an area of congestion or oedema to an area with functioning lymphatics.

mastectomy Surgical removal of most of the breast tissue.

microsurgery Surgery using a microscope and computer-guided instruments, often employed to join small lymph or blood vessels.

musculature The muscular apparatus of the body or a body part.

myxoedema A special form of oedema associated with impairment of the thyroid gland, generally resulting from an accumulation of mucinoid substances in the tissues.

oedema The presence of abnormally large amounts of fluid in the spaces between the cells, which produces swelling.

parathyroid glands Four small glands attached to the thyroid glands and located below the larynx, which control the level of calcium in the body.

phlebo-lymphoedema Oedema of the legs and feet caused by damage to the lymphatic system owing to chronic insufficiency of the veins.

primary lymphoedema *See* lymphoedema.

proximal Nearest to the centre of the body or the point of attachment.

radiotherapy Treatment of disease by means of X-rays or radioactive substances.

sebaceous glands Glands in the skin which secrete an oily substance that keeps the skin smooth and supple.

sebum The oily secretion of the sebaceous glands.

secondary lymphoedema *See* lymphoedema.

sentinel lymph node The first lymph node that drains from a tumour.

spleen A large, gland-like organ in the upper left part of the abdomen, which filters the blood. It is one of the sites where lymphocytes are formed.

streptococcus A type of bacteria usually ocurring in pairs or chains.

subcutaneous Located just below the skin.

thrombosis The development of a clot in a blood vessel.

thymus A small organ in the upper chest, where lymphocytes mature. It is an important part of the immune system.

thyroid gland The largest of the endocrine glands, located in the neck. It produces hormones that are important for the body's growth and metabolic processes.

tonometry A diagnostic technique for measuring the resistance of lymphatic tissue to compression, which indicates the amount of fibrosis present.

tonsils Two small masses of lymphatic tissue at the back of the throat.

tracer material Radioactive material which can be followed usually by means of a gamma camera.

ultrasound A technique used to create an image of soft tissue by bouncing sound waves off the part of the body under investigation.

valve A mechanism which ensures that fluids in the lymph and blood vessels flow only in one direction.

varicose Veins or arteries abnormally distended.

vascular system The network of vessels that carries blood around the body.

venous Associated with the veins or blood system.